The Theta Way

Health & Wellness Through Science & Technology

Kristine Dohner
Janet Garland

Copyright ©2023 by Kristine Dohner & Janet Garland

All rights reserved. No part of this publication may be reproduced, stored in a retrieval system, or transmitted in any form or by any means – for example, electronic, mechanical, recording, or photocopying, without the prior written consent of the authors. The only exception is brief quotations in printed reviews.

Note – Important: The information contained in this book is for educational purposes only. Any medical condition discussed should be diagnosed/cared for under the direction of a physician. This book is not designed to diagnose, treat, or prescribe any disease. The authors accept no responsibility for such use. The ideas and suggestions herein are our own experiences. There may be some ideas in the book that may not agree with orthodox, allopathic medicine.

Throughout the book, we have shared stories that others have shared with us about their "Theta Way" experiences using the equipment, modalities, and protocols we write about. While we have made great effort to present accurate recollections, the names have been changed for client privacy.

Published by Kristine Dohner & Janet Garland

Kristinedohner@gmail.com
JanetG.Theta@gmail.com
www.ThetaWellnessCenterInc.com

Cover Design: Jaime Partlow

ISBN: 9798391374886

"When you have exhausted all possibilities, remember this - you haven't."

- Thomas Edison

CONTENTS

	PREFACE	ix
	INTRODUCTION	xiii
1	WHAT IS HAPPENING IN THE WORLD TODAY?	1
	In the Beginning...	3
2	THE SCIENCE OF FREQUENCY	7
	The Science of Frequency is Not New	7
	Early Days of Frequency Science	9
	Body Frequency	10
3	WHAT IS THE THETA WAY?	13
	What Defines Us	13
	How Theta Wellness Technology Began	14
4	IF YOU WANT SOMETHING DIFFERENT, YOU MUST DO SOMETHING DIFFERENT	19
	ThetaChamber℠	21
	Vestibular Motion	23
	Binaural Audio Beats	25
	Cranial Electronic Stimulation	26
	Visual Light Pattern Stimulation	29
	Hyper-Cube Hyperbaric Oxygen Therapy	32
	How It Benefits the Body	32
	Facts & Benefits of Low-Pressure Hyperbaric Therapy	33
	LED Light Therapy Bed	36
	AO Scan Digital Analyzer	41
	Repetitive Transcranial Magnetic Stimulation (rTMS)	51
5	HEALTH & WELLNESS THROUGH SCIENCE & TECHNOLOGY	55
	Acoustic Light Wave	55
	Hydrogen Therapy	57
	Presso-Therapy	59
	Radio Frequency (RF) Detox	60
	Vibration (Vibe) Plate	62
	Brainspotting Trauma Therapy	64

6	**EMOTIONAL & MENTAL HEALTH**	69
	Addiction/Substance Abuse	70
	Depression	76
	Post-Traumatic Stress Disorder (PTSD)	78
	Stress & Anxiety	81
	Insomnia	85
	Attention Deficit Disorder (ADD)/Attention Deficit Hyperactivity Disorder (ADHD)/Oppositional Defiance Disorder (ODD)	88
	Executive Tune-Up	90
	Neuropathy	91
	Pain Management	92
	Concentration, Focus, & Memory	93
	Athletic Edge	94
	Boosted Immunity	96
	Whole-Body Detox	97
	Tune-Up Station	98
7	**HEALTH BEGINS IN THE GUT**	101
	Why the Gut is So Important	101
	Problems with the Standard American Diet	102
	Other Causes of Poor Gut Health	103
	The Brain-Gut Connection	106
	Metals, Molds, Pollutants, & Pesticides	107
	We Offer Resources…	109
	Negative Ion H_2O Sticks	109
	Theta Chamber	109
	AO Digital Body Analyzer Scan	110
	Inner Voice	111
	Vitals Scan	111
	Comprehensive Scan	112
	ACKNOWLEDGMENTS	115
	ABOUT THE AUTHORS	117

> *"The limits of the possible can only be defined by going beyond them into the impossible."*
>
> — Arthur C. Clarke

The Theta Way

PREFACE

Janet

In 2018, I visited the Innergy Development, Inc. headquarters as a fun field trip during a reunion trip with my four sisters. Our goal at these annual get-togethers is always to enjoy each other's company while we explore an area and experience something new. We all had AO Scan Digital Body Analysis done and then tried out several pieces of the equipment. We were so incredibly relaxed and had such positive experiences that we went back for more treatments. At first, I was just curious about the equipment and machinery.

Over our days together, we shared our stories and experiences with different modalities: we were all pretty amazed. The sister who had arranged for us to go had previously used the LED Light Bed, which helped her with post-surgery recovery. Not only did we have a fun experience, we all felt terrific from using the equipment.

During our stay, I was able to meet the company's owner, Loran Swensen, who designed and manufactured the equipment. We heard the history behind each piece of equipment's design and about the people those protocols had helped - it was awe-inspiring. My own experience started me on the path of understanding the science and theory of the Theta Way. I got excited that there was technology that could help people beyond traditional (allopathic) medicine. Machines that used cutting-edge brain science were able to help people in safe and non-invasive ways.

I witnessed Loran and his staff's passion for the equipment, the stories, and the successes over the years of those who came through their clinics. I knew I wanted to be part of this history in the making and bring it to my community and to Northern California. Through the Theta Wellness Center in Gold River, I have genuinely seen lives changed, and health improved. I have witnessed people entering the facility in a frail or depressed state and then leaving feeling strong, full of life, and ready to take on new challenges. We have served all ages, from three weeks old to those closer to the century mark.

In opening up and running our Theta Wellness Center, I have been fortunate to gather some of the kindest, brightest, and most thoughtful staff. They carry my same desire: to bring hope and support to suffering, hurting people on their journey toward healing and wholeness.

Theta technology is the way of the future, and it is here now. Every day when I arrive at the center, I am excited about the opportunity to bring positive, healing change to the lives of others. This book includes some of those success stories with the hope that you may be encouraged in your journey to health and well-being.

Kristine

In addition to working with Janet, I have the good fortune of being her sister. I was at the same reunion where we five sisters experienced the Theta Way. Our needs and experiences were varied, even though we are genetically from the same tree. I love the technology we offer and how we can use proven science to help and support people who, like us, have diverse challenges. We have been able to witness transformation before our very eyes. But perhaps my greatest joy is hearing every person's story, which is as unique as they are. Science is great, but, to me, seeing lives and relationships healed and improved is even better.

At the Theta Wellness Center, I am often busy doing Brainspotting, trauma therapy, and, occasionally, AO Scan Digital full-body scans. As an ordained pastor, it is very satisfying to help people spiritually and support their souls and body. I believe God cares deeply about all three, and the abundant life He promises comes through the wholeness of the spirit, soul, and body.

I have been asked how I reconcile my Christian beliefs with the science and technology of alternative healing methods. To me, its not either/or; all wisdom comes from the Creator, who spoke existence into being (frequency and sound) and that creative power is still going forth.

My motivation for writing this book comes from a desire to let people know about the brain science, technology, and practical helps we offer through the Theta Wellness Center. For many who seek us out, we are the "last resort" after they have tried traditional avenues of healing, convinced there must be something more. While we don't make promises, people who come to the center often comment that, at the very least, they feel seen, heard, and cared for. That in itself can be very healing.

You likely picked up this book because you are on your own unique healing journey. Whether or not we ever have the blessing of meeting you in person, we wish you the best possible outcome. May you find what you are looking for.

*"There are only two ways to live your life.
One is as though nothing is a miracle.
The other is as though everything is a miracle."*
                                        - Albert Einstein

INTRODUCTION

Why are we writing this book?

Every experience we have as human beings result from our brain waves: the electrical impulses in the brain. Neurons within our brains communicate our behavior, emotions, and thoughts. As your brain goes, so, too, will you.

There is science and technology available in leading-edge, non-invasive (no instruments introduced into the body and no skin broken) modalities that, when used individually or in sequence, can create a positive change in an individual's life. For people aged newborn to 90s or older, these modalities can help improve or reverse the limitations they are currently living with. In this book, we introduce you to what makes a Theta Wellness Center unique: how different modalities, proven by science, research, and time, can change physical and mental outcomes for people seeking a way to "live their best life."

The world is ever-changing; we are affected daily by the science within our bodies and all around us. Brain Science and Alternative Wellness technologies are available to support you on your journey to optimal health and wellness. This book contains information about time-honored scientific studies where outcomes have been successful and stories of client success in managing and supporting common health issues.

You don't have to look far to see that health and wholeness are on the hearts and minds of people, now more than ever. You can't get very far down a street without seeing health food stores, gyms, yoga studios, IV (intravenous) therapy centers, counseling services, mental health facilities, substance abuse centers, and more in neighborhoods all over. We want health, and we need wholeness. Many new medical innovations, holistic methodologies, preventive measures, positive thinking, and behavior modification are available. Yet, the Center for Disease Control (CDC) reports that life expectancy in the United States is at its lowest since 2003. (77.3 years)[1]

Some urgent pursuits for health and preventive health are likely because chronic and life-threatening diseases (including heart disease, cancer, and diabetes) are at an all-time high. They touch everyone: it's almost certain you know someone, know of someone, or know someone who knows someone that suffers from one or more. The American Cancer Society estimated in 2021, there would be 1,898,160 new cancer cases and 608,570 cancer deaths in the United States. That works out to 5,200 new cases of cancer each day and 1,600 deaths per day.[2] In his book *Life Force*, Tony Robbins writes that cancer is so commonplace that 40 percent of Americans can expect to receive a diagnosis at some point.

To find out how vital well-being is to people today, you need only follow the money. In addition to traditional medicine,

---

[1] Elizabet Arias, Ph.D., Betzaida Tejada-Vera, M.S., Farida Ahmad, P.P.H., and Kenneth D. Kochanek, M.A., NVSS, *Vital Statistics Rapid Release Report* No. 015, July 2021

[2] CA: *A Cancer Journal for Clinicians*, https://acsjournals.onlinelibrary.wiley.com/doi/full/10.3322/caac.21654

which is a multi-trillion-dollar per year industry, the alternative medicine industry revenue has grown to over 21 billion dollars annually in the United States. Alternative medicine refers to any form of treatment or protocol outside the mainstream of conventional (allopathic) medicine, as practiced by most physicians, clinics, and hospitals. Well-known examples include osteopathy, acupuncture, and homeopathy[3].

In addition to obesity, it is increasingly more common for young people to suffer from "older people" problems: kidney stones, Type-2 diabetes, high cholesterol, and hypertension. Poor diet, lack of exercise, and sedentary lifestyle are easy to blame. Regardless of the reasons, it is sad that this generation is the first generation that will live sicker and die younger than previous generations. Millennials (born between 1981 and 1995) are seeing their health decline faster than the previous generation - both physical and behavioral health conditions. The report suggests that without intervention, millennials could see mortality rates climb by more than 40% compared to Gen-Xers (born between 1965-1980) at the same age.[4]

So, health is an all-important topic for all ages; we think about it, learn about it, and invest in it. We live in the days of instant "Dr. Google" and WebMD, where everyone can access facts and information at their fingertips. Even so, public perception is building that we can find health in healing tools beyond traditional medicine. We have been drugged and regimented, but those methods have not always gotten deep enough to the

---

[3] Matej Mikulic, Estimated Alternative medicine industry revenue in the U.S. from 2011 to 2021, https://statista.com/stistics/203972/alternative-medicine-revenue-growth/, October 25, 2021

[4] *The Economic Consequences of Millennial Health,* Moody's Analytics, Blue Cross Blue Shield: The Health of America, November 16, 2019

core to make the changes necessary to help sustain a healthy lifestyle. While neither inherently bad nor unnecessary, the medical and pharmaceutical world does not often support alternative means when it takes profit out of their pockets.

Declining health is a trend that shows no signs of slowing or reversing. So, what can you do? It is said, "If You Want Something Different, You Must Do Something Different."

*"If you want to find the secrets of the universe,
think in terms of energy, vibration, and frequency."*
— Nikola Tesla

1 WHAT IS HAPPENING IN THE WORLD TODAY?

We are currently living in the far-reaching aftermath of the Covid-19 pandemic. The World Health Organization reports that the health crisis killed people, spread human suffering, and upended people's lives worldwide. But, more than a health crisis, it was a human, economic, and social crisis, as it attacked societies at their core.[5] Negative psychological effects include post-traumatic stress symptoms, confusion, fear, and anger. Stressors include infection, fears, frustration, boredom, inadequate supplies, inadequate/inaccurate information, financial loss, death of loved ones, and stigma.

Many organizations report increases in insomnia, eating difficulties, and increases in alcohol consumption or substance abuse: all due to worry and stress. The World Health Organization in March 2022, reported that anxiety and depression had increased worldwide by over 25% in the prior two years. The faces of suicide victims and those attempting suicide were younger and more numerous than at any recent time in history. A generation of babies was born into a society of mask requirements. Even after relaxed restrictions, many are

---

[5]Everyone Included: Social Impact of Covid-19,
https://www.un.org/development/desa/dspd/everyone-included-covid-19.html

afraid to go "mask free" as they feel uncomfortable without something on their face. In short, people have been traumatized and are unsure how to reach a "normal" state.

> *"Trauma is perhaps the most avoided, ignored, belittled, denied, misunderstood, and untreated cause of human suffering."*
> - Peter A. Levine, PhD

Trauma is not a new malady. An estimated 90% of adults in the United States have experienced a traumatic event at least once; eight million people have post-traumatic stress disorder (PTSD) at any given time. Specific groups (such as first responders) have an even higher concentration of those numbers.[6]

One attorney we know said that during the pandemic, his firm's divorce caseload increased so much they could not keep up with the demand. In short, people are scared, sick, anxious, lonely, sad, hopeless, and traumatized. Now, more than ever, it may be the time to utilize new science to tackle both old and new problems. Where do we start?

Let's begin with understanding the body better. Everything has a vibration; everything living moves. Nothing in life is without movement. The atoms which make up everything are in a constant state of motion. The speed of these atoms will determine whether things appear as solid, liquid, or gas. The entire material world is nothing but vibration: sound is a vibration, and so are colors and thoughts - all living things have frequency and vibration. In addition to your need for air, water, and nutrition, your body is a fantastic machine that runs on energy and requires maintenance and calibration.

---

[6] Bessel A. van der Kolk, MD, *The Body Keeps Score: Brain, Mind, and Body in the Healing of Trauma*, Penguin Books, 2014

Energy, frequency, vibration, and resonance are the four keys that unlock energetic well-being. The speed or rate at which something vibrates is its frequency. The only difference between one object and another is the rate of its vibration or vibrational frequency. Every cell of your body produces energy. The frequencies involve the movement of energy from your cells to the brain and back. Through this line of communication, over 120,000 blueprint frequencies (tones and frequencies in the healthy range) travel at a consistent rate and speed in healthy bodies.

When energy is too low, you feel sluggish and muddled. When energy is too high, you feel hyper and chaotic. When energy is just right, you feel your body running according to design. Each cell broadcasts a unique vibratory sound signature describing everything going on inside. When parts of the body become stressed or diseased, they no longer produce the correct sound wave nor operate at their optimal frequency. The harmony of those frequencies in your body significantly affects your overall health and well-being. In recalibrating your frequency, it's helpful to understand how lower and higher vibrations affect your energy and health.

In the beginning...

In humankind's early history, there were only naturally-occurring frequencies and sounds (vibrations). As tools and products developed and the world moved toward industrialization, manufactured sound, vibration, and frequency increased and were released into the atmosphere. Toxic byproducts made their way into the air, the water, the soil, and our food supply. Little did we know miracle weedkillers could cause debilitating and fatal effects down the road. Neither did we know, when mining and working with heavy metals, that toxins and metals could pass down for several generations in the blood through the umbilical cord. This is called a transgenerational effect.[7]

Today, you can make very healthy food and lifestyle choices but still be affected by what continues to exist around you. You can grow a clean, organic garden, but if your neighbor's yard is not pesticide-free, your yard may not be completely organic. Wind and insects can cross-contaminate. Living in an area with no industry, you may still breathe air tainted by fuel, and toxins spewed into the air of urban regions.

Every day, you are exposed to noise and frequency: lights, electricity, power lines, machinery, engines, appliances, HVAC systems, television and radio, computers, and other running mechanical devices. When a sound wave travels outward from its source, it spreads like a wave when a stone drops in water: continuing to spread out over time.

The wave pattern formed by different vibrations would look like a series of overlaying, concentric circles moving into each other.[8] Those circles of exposure will affect your body over time. Logic says that if those frequencies are constructive, they could benefit your well-being. Suppose those vibrations are the same (constructive) as your body's rhythm. In that case, the effect strengthens and amplifies the frequency. Frequencies oppositional (destructive) to your body's rhythm could be damaging over time.

---

[7] https://www.ewg.org/research/how-toxic-pollutants-can-harm-future-unexposed-generations
[8] http:Sciencelearn.org.nz/resources/2816-sound-wave-interference, September 13, 2019

Just as sound and frequency can affect your body negatively, the intentional use of specific frequencies can bring you to a more balanced version of yourself. The science of sound, frequency, and vibration utilized for health and well-being is not new. Science and technology offer healthy frequencies to help us get our bodies back to homeostasis (the ability to maintain internal stability to compensate for environmental changes).

*"Impossibility only lasts until you find
new unbelievable hard evidence."*
— Toba Beta

2 THE SCIENCE OF FREQUENCY

The Science of Frequency is Not New

Science and innovation are areas where we stand on the shoulders of inventors and scientists that have gone before us. We sit in chairs daily without considering who first developed the design. Over time, chairs have gone from simple, crude construction to high-end, custom-fitted, ergonomically-designed models.

The same is true for frequency, light, and vibration science. Over the years, discovery and progress in design have enabled forward movement with more sophisticated ways to harness and utilize what was once a simple discovery. Historically, new discoveries have often encountered strong resistance within the medical community. Anything challenging current methods and practices has been met with the innovator being discredited, black-listed, and financially or vocationally crushed by their contemporaries.

When hand and instrument washing between patients was first introduced to the medical community by Dr. Ignaz Semmelweis in 1846, doctors rejected it. They wore blood on their lab coats as a badge of importance and accomplishment. Dr. Semmelweis, trying to decrease deaths in maternity wards of perpetual fever known as childbed fever, ordered his medical staff to start cleaning their hands and instruments, not with just soap, but with a chlorine solution (still one of the most effective disinfectants). Knowing nothing about germs, he figured it would at least eliminate any smell left behind from the last procedure.

Dr. Semmelweis discovered what we now know as common knowledge: handwashing is a critical tool in public health. Nurses and midwives started the new hygiene practice immediately, and patient mortalities took a drastic, noticeable decline. (The doctors, upset because it made it look like they were the ones giving childbed fever to the women, refused to wash their hands; their spread of disease and high patient mortality rates continued.) Semmelweis was criticized, humiliated, and his discoveries were ignored.

Later, the germ theory was discovered (the idea that microorganisms we can't even see cause certain diseases and infections). The existence of germs is now an "of course." Today, as then, there are pressures from institutions and money-making organizations to squelch anything that does not financially benefit them. It is not difficult to see why so many amazing discoveries have initially been "thrown under the bus."

In 19th century Germany, Heinrich Rudolf Hertz was the first scientist to prove the existence of electromagnetic waves. He utilized procedures and designed instruments to generate and detect waves (radio pulses) across space. He demonstrated that all forms of electromagnetic radiation are continued or increased at the speed of light. In recognition of his significant discoveries, Hertz's name is the universal synonym for frequency. The term Hz (pronounced "Hertz") refers to the number of cycles per second, which we know as frequency.

Hertz's discoveries about frequency became the launching pad for many medical and media technologies. Today, many modern comforts and scientific tools are built upon Hertz's research and experiments. These include radio waves, microwaves, infrared, optical, ultraviolet, x-ray, and gamma rays – all measured in Hz.[9]

Early Days of Frequency Science

Nikola Tesla was one of the most fascinating and prolific electrical inventors of the late nineteenth and early twentieth centuries. A Serbian American inventor and engineer, he discovered and patented the rotating magnetic field, the basis of most alternating-current machinery, the three-phase electric power transmission system, oscillators, meters, improved lights, experimented with x-rays, and designed the high voltage coil known as the Tesla coil, widely used in radio technology. Tesla, Inc., a well-known American manufacturer of electric automobiles, solar panels, and batteries for cars and home storage, was named as a nod to Nikola Tesla's ground-breaking discoveries. As with many early inventors, Tesla was unable to turn his genius into significant personal financial gain.

Albert Einstein was the first to state, "The future of medicine is frequency." He was one of the most brilliant people ever to be born and won worldwide fame for his theory of relativity (considered controversial then.) Einstein won a Nobel Prize in 1921 for explaining Hertz's photoelectric effect. He built on Hertz's theories to form the science of cosmology (the universe is dynamic instead of static, capable of expanding and contracting). He made important contributions to developing the theory of quantum mechanics, a pillar of modern physics.

---

[9] Patricia Spieth Ramsay, *Heinrich Hertz, the Father of Frequency*, https://pubmed.ncbinlm.gov/2682537, March 2013

Royal Raymond Rife discovered that specific radio frequencies, when broadcast through a plasma tube towards the body, would only affect microbes that resonated that exact frequency. And when that frequency hits a microbe, it destroys that specific microbe, having absolutely no effect on anything else.

Rife discovered that a specific set of frequencies could be broadcast through the air around us. In the same way, we broadcast cell phone calls, radio, and television signals today; they affect only the intended target. It's like shooting a fly with a laser beam versus a shotgun: while they can both take out the fly, the laser beam leaves everything else in tack.

Our technology today was once just a dream. It is important to keep an open mind regarding things we don't yet understand. The research, design, exploration, and experiments today will bring essential answers to the health needs of future generations.

Body Frequency

What Tesla, Einstein, and others once theorized, scientific researchers from Harvard and NASA are rapidly discovering. The body is a complex electromagnetic field of energy waves that serve as "control central" for our physical and mental well-being. Scientists uncovered that the entire world is full of electric currents and magnetic fields, challenging entrenched thinking in biology. Natural and manufactured frequencies surrounding us affect and change human cells. Wellness can come from positively manipulating the energy that flows through our bodies to reach a state of homeostasis.

Every living thing vibrates at a particular frequency: molecules, cells, tissues, organs, parasites, bacteria, viruses, etc. A healthy heart, for example, will continuously vibrate at a particular frequency regardless of age, weight, height, stature, or ethos. Frequencies work like guitar strings: how tight or loose the strings are strung will determine the tone the guitar gives off. Change the tension and you change the tone. Imbalances, disorders, and diseases alter the frequency of the body's "bioenergetic communication" network (the guitar strings); balancing frequency can help your body heal itself. Bringing the body's systems back into the healthy range of tone and frequency, known as "blueprint frequencies," enables you to gain better health and retain healing.

"The future of medicine is frequency."
— Albert Einstein

3 WHAT IS THE THETA WAY?

What Defines Us

The Theta Way refers to cutting-edge technologies and modalities that utilize "theta" science to optimize health and well-being. Theta Wellness Center offers innovative new tools that optimize frequency balance in the human body. We have a database of over 120,000 time-tested and proven blueprint frequencies that define normal frequency in the human body. Our therapies focus on adjusting frequencies that are out of balance to prevent dysfunction and boost vitality. It is like getting a powerful tune-up.

At our Theta Wellness Center here in Gold River, you can experience the latest light, vibrational and electromagnetic interventions. These include Pulse Electromagnetic Field (PEMF) therapy, vibrational plates, red and infrared light treatment, altitude barometric therapy, oxygen therapy, hydrogen therapy, and pulse brain stimulation. We incorporate interventions into our electromagnetic, bio-sonic, and bio-photonic fields that we believe will create entirely new approaches, new products, and business models.

Theta Wellness Center offers the core group of Theta-Chamber^{SM}, rTMS (Repetitive Transcranial Magnetic Stimulation) unit, an LED Light Bed, and a Hyperbaric Cube (oxygen chamber). Additionally, individual centers have various supplementary equipment to support and reinforce the healing process. At our center, we additionally offer the AO Scan Digital Analyzer, Inner Hydrogen therapy, Vibration (Vibe) Plate, Acoustic Light Wave (based on RIFE frequencies), RF (radio frequency) Innergy Detox, Presso-Therapy, IV therapy, Erectile Dysfunction therapy, Vaginal and Urethral/bladder Rejuvenation, Cosmetic-Youthful Facial Therapy, Brainspotting trauma therapy, Pain Management, and Nutritional counseling.

These terms and concepts may seem unfamiliar, but we will help you understand the science of these machines, modalities, and descriptions of how each works in this book.

How Theta Wellness Technology Began

Loran Swensen, the founder of Innergy Development Inc. in Provo, Utah, shares the story of his journey that resulted in the creation and design of the ThetaChamber[SM]:

"We adopted our son, Michael, at nine months old, and he came with a pre-existing condition called cerebral palsy. We were new parents and just delighted to have him in our lives. As Michael grew over the next few years, his cerebral palsy became more and more evident. By the time he started preschool, about four or five years old, he walked with his arms over his head, kind of bouncing off the walls to maintain his balance. So, it was evident that he was heading in that direction, that a wheelchair would be coming up soon.

"Like any parents, we just wanted Michael to have the best life possible. So, we traveled all around looking for therapies for children with cerebral palsy. We wanted to improve his quality of life. Everywhere we went within the United States we were met with the same explanation, 'There is no cure for Cerebral Palsy. The best we offer is diet and exercise to improve his quality of life.' As parents, that wasn't good enough. We believed there had to be something better. And when we went outside of the country: Mexico, Germany, and one trip to Japan, there was more hope there; more therapies available. That encouraged me to look in different directions.

"This was back in the 1980s when the internet wasn't around. So, we went to trade shows and health fairs. I was introduced to a book called *Mega Brain* by Michael Hutchins, and that book became my new bible when it came to therapies for Michael. Through that book, I came across treatments presented by Dr. David Clark, Ohio State University of Medicine, Dr. Margaret "Meg" Patterson, a surgeon out of Aberdeen, Scotland, and Dr. Michael Persinger at Laurentian University in Toronto, Canada. These three doctors had been pioneering different therapies; they didn't know anything about each other.

"Dr. Clark was working with spinning a child in a chair to help develop the inner ear. They found that this was helping with all sorts of neurological issues. Dr. Persinger used different flashing lights to stimulate the right and left brain connections. Dr. Patterson applied a microcurrent right behind the ear or to the earlobe to create new neural pathways. These three things were pretty important to me. So, as we looked into this, we developed a machine that later became known as the ThetaChamber℠. Michael was the first recipient of this technology. When Michael began, he was eight years old, and his Cerebral Palsy was increasingly becoming an issue in his mobility. It was a 21-day course of action based on what Doctors Persinger, Clark, and Patterson were doing.

"At the end of 21 days, we saw some improvement: he was processing information faster, and there was some improvement in his mobility. The next six months were magical as his mobility became normal. He also transitioned from a special needs school to a mainstream school. Michael is now 40, a second-degree black belt, speaks multiple languages, and physically you would never know that Michael had Cerebral Palsy.

"That whole experience was life-changing for our family. I realized that there were things we didn't know here, which led me on the journey to where we are today in 2023. We learned about frequencies, different therapies, our belief systems, what we say to ourselves, and how all these things affect us.

"In 2008, my wife and I were attending a medical convention in China. There was a booth there from Russia where they had developed a scanner that scanned the body in frequency. That was a significant area of interest for me. We experienced a digital body scan in the booth with these big transducers on our heads, and it nailed us! It showed everything wrong or awry in our bodies. We later worked with that company and acquired the rights to bring it to the United States.

"We did that until 2012 when technology advanced (Windows 10 became available), and we realized software would not be stable. It was written in the late 1980s and early 1990s and was no longer supported. The company had decided to bag it; they said we were pretty much on our own. We rewrote all that software for the next two to three years into today's platform and technology. We came up with what is now the AO Scan Digital Body Scanner.

"It was a big system, a $30,000 machine that would sit in a doctor's office and take one to three hours, depending on the scan. We improved it to use much smaller transducers, and a scan can now be completed in 45 minutes to an hour. Part of that scanner is Inner Voice, where we record 10-20 seconds of your voice and analyze 2,000 frequencies over 12 notes. We are looking for frequencies that are out of range: too high or very low. We send you balancing frequencies for those currently out of balance. Listening to those frequencies played back in your headset helps with those emotions and helps with some of the physical issues you've been dealing with. We thought that would be an amazing tool to get into as many hands as possible. When you can get your emotions under control, you can have a better physical outcome."

The use of frequency instruments has been around for over a century. We just don't always think of these instruments as frequency devices: electro-cauterization units, electric scalpels, pulsed short-wave diathermy used for deep tissue heating, TENS units, ultrasound units, Bio-Feedback devices, lasers used for other treatments, such as acne and weight reduction are all frequency devices.

"Everything is theoretically impossible until it is done."
- Robert A. Heinlein

4 IF YOU WANT SOMETHING DIFFERENT, YOU MUST DO SOMETHING DIFFERENT

"You never change your life until you step out of your comfort zone; change begins at the end of your comfort zone."

- Roy T. Bennett

Many people can easily relate to this quote. We all had things we needed to go above and beyond to achieve. Sometimes that requires doing something completely different than we have ever done, which necessitates stepping outside our comfort zone - and some level of bravery. It's not easy to tell yourself to do more or to do something you have never done before, bravely. But what if that very thing is a key to your healing? Perhaps Thomas Jefferson said it best, "If you want something you have never had, you must be willing to do something you have never done."

Doing only what you know and usually do has gotten you to where you are today. If you want more, you need to do more or something different. That is where significant accomplishments are achieved, inventions are created, records are broken, and breakthrough happens.

Can some machines help you get healthier, smarter, more capable or creative, less stressed, more relaxed, and better able to rest and sleep? Yes! The development of brain-exploring technology has become front and center in brain research, involving scientists from psychology to neuroscience. Ideas and processes that sounded like "strange voodoo" even a decade ago are now widely accepted and credible.

Just as regular exercise creates strength and benefits for the body, we now have machines and devices that stimulate brain growth and development. We shared earlier that as the brain goes, so goes the body. It was once believed that the total number of brain cells we have was completed by age two; that no matter what experiences or stimulations the brain receives, the number of brain cells could not increase. Dr. Amar Sahay, a neuroscientist with Harvard-affiliated Massachusetts General Hospital, says, "The dogma for the longest time was that adult brains couldn't generate any new brain cells. You just use what you were born with, but the reality is that everyone has the capacity to develop new cells that can enhance cognitive functions."[10]

You can develop new brain cells, and you can try new things. People who are set in their ways, who resist any new idea, who hate to try something new, who refer to and relive every experience and idea from their past, who must always be right and never experience the stimulation and self-doubt of something new, cut off the influx of new energy from their brain. They may feel self-satisfied but experience lower levels of mental connectedness and complexity. They get stuck in a rut. If that describes you, now is a great time to address it.

---

[10] http://www.health.harvard.edu/mind-and-mood/can-you-grow-new-brain-cells, September 14, 2016

Forward movement is difficult if you follow the same routines day after day. Why not make today the first day of your new life?

"Your attitude plus your choices equals your life."
- Anonymous

The ThetaChamber℠

The modern ThetaChamber℠ is the state-of-the-art version of a chamber that was originally developed by Loran Swensen (pictured to the left) in 1989, called the Omega Brain 5000.

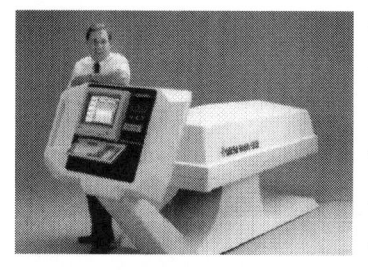

The central feature of the Theta Wellness Center is the Theta-Chamber℠. It is designed to induce a person's brainwave activity into a wavelength scientifically referred to as the theta brain wave state. This is the state of relaxation that is well known as the drowsy, abstract sensation that one feels as they are drifting into a deep sleep. In the theta rhythm (4-7 Hz), the mind is capable of deep and profound learning, healing, and growth.

In this state, the brain is no longer focused on sensory perception but on the subconscious, where new mental patterns form as the brain processes information. The ThetaChamber℠ administers powerful treatment applications in a single session with our three main objectives:

1. Induce a theta brain wave state, opening the brain to learning, healing, and growth.
2. Signal the hypothalamus to return to producing normal levels of serotonin, dopamine, and other neurotransmitters.
3. Encourage the brain to create and use new neural pathways.

The ThetaChamber℠ technology represents a break-through in the treatment of neurological issues:

Depression	Parkinson's Disease
ADD/ADHD/OCD	Learning Enhancement
Anxiety/Stress	Chronic Pain
Insomnia	Memory, Focus, &
PTSD	Concentration
Addiction: Drugs/Alcohol/ Gaming/Pornography/Sugar…	

Stress, anxiety, depression, addiction, and mental illness are among the most alarming and fastest-growing epidemics today. The ThetaChamber℠ is a unique breakthrough in personal development that helps the brain to reduce stress and regain chemical balance.

The chamber delivers a highly therapeutic effect using subtle and non-invasive modalities, such as vestibular motion, binaural beats, cranial-electrotherapy stimulation, and visual light pattern stimulation. Many clients report that time in the ThetaChamber℠ is more relaxing than a massage.

Clients initially feel an enhanced sense of time and space as the chamber begins its spin. The lights, beats, and subtle currents serve as sensory stimulation, delivering customized frequencies.

Then the person feels deep relaxation and a stimulation of specific brain activities. Many have experienced profound, moving experiences, allowing them to escape their dark cycle of difficulty at first momentarily and, ultimately, for good.

Due to the great success in helping clients overcome stress, depression, anxiety, addiction, etc., through their sense and volition, the ThetaChamber[SM] has become available for integration with other therapies such as psychiatry, counseling, life coaching, and addiction recovery working in tandem with depression/stress management clinics, doctor's offices, and holistic healing centers.

Vestibular Motion

The ThetaChamber[SM] spins! Vestibular motion is a direct result of NASA research. Astronauts are subjected to spinning and rocking movements so that they will become accustomed to the feelings and movement in outer space. The vestibular system is a sensory system that creates a sense of balance and spatial orientation for the purpose of coordinating movement with balance. The liquid level in our inner ear and individual vestibular components send signals to accomplish this task.

The spinning of the ThetaChamber[SM] throws off the brain's natural sense of time and space, all while enhancing the flow of the person's bio-magnetic field. The spinning causes the inner ear to balance and gives off a sense of floating, which relaxes the body.

The chamber synchronizes in speed (13 rpm) and direction with the Earth's natural rotation, so you don't feel the spin. Disrupting the brain's tracking of time and space allows activity to stimulate atrophied parts of the brain. With Autism clients, the chamber spins at the same speed as the Earth's rotation but in the opposite direction.

People who spend 30 minutes in the ThetaChamber[SM] pod usually report feeling like they are floating or rocking, losing time. While many clients are initially concerned about feeling the spin or claustrophobia, it is rare for anyone to stop their treatment early. All of the equipment has a panic button the client can quickly push that immediately stops and opens the machine. All ages can benefit from ThetaChamber[SM] modalities, including infants, children, and babies in utero.

Numerous studies have shown vestibular stimulation to affect brain development, integration, intelligence, and behavior modification. The following is a sample of the effects reported in literature:

- Developmentally delayed children displayed significant advances in speech development after vestibular stimulation treatment.[11]
- Children exposed to vestibular stimulation showed significant improvement in gross motor skills.[12]
- Vestibular stimulation made impressive improvements in the behavior of children diagnosed with ADHD. Improvement persisted throughout the follow-up one year later.[13]

---

[11] Magrun M, et. Al., *Effects of Vestibular Stimulation on Spontaneous Use of Verbal Language in Developmentally Delayed Children*, American Journal of Occupational Therapy, 2:101-104, 1981

[12] Clark DL et. Al., *Vestibular Stimulation Influence on Motor Development in Infants*, Science, 10 June 1977, Vol. 196 no. 4295:1228-1229

[13] Arnold LE t. al. Vestibular and Visual Rotational Stimulation as Treatment for

Binaural Audio Beats

Subtle pulses or "beats" are created when slightly offset tones play through headphones, which brings the brain into a theta state. Utilizing bilateral stimulation enables both sides of the brain to interact and communicate with each other. Bilateral stimulation is believed to bypass the area of the brain that gets stuck in trauma, unhealthy habits, or addiction and prevent the brain's left side from self-soothing the right side of the brain.

Heinrich Wilhelm Dove discovered this effect in 1839. The impact on brainwaves depends on the difference in frequencies of each tone. For example, if 315 Hz was played in one ear and 325 in the other, the binaural beat would have a frequency of 10 Hz. The beats synchronize the brain hemispheres and help produce the right conditions for neural pathway re-establishment, also known as "entrainment." The result is deep relaxation.

Research in 2019 of 22 studies found that binaural beats reduced anxiety. A 2007 study from the National College of Medicine in Oregon showed that binaural beats decreased anxiety and increased IGF and dopamine.[14]

Attention Deficit and hyperactivity, American Journal of Occupational Therapy, 39, 84-91, 1985

[14] Helane' Wahbeh, Carlo Calabrese, Heather Zwickey, *Binaural beat technology in humans: a pilot study to access psychologic and physiologic affects*, National Library of Medicine, 2007, Jan-Feb, 13(1), 25-32

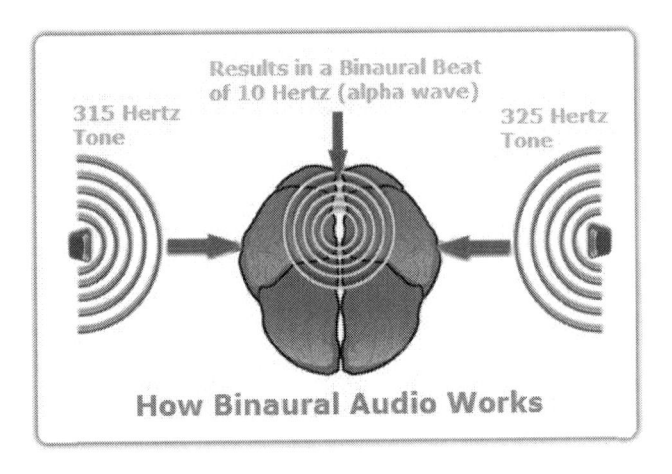

315 Hertz Tone — Results in a Binaural Beat of 10 Hertz (alpha wave) — **325 Hertz Tone**

How Binaural Audio Works

Cranial Electrotherapy Stimulation (CES)

CES uses micro-current stimulation and is a primary modality utilized in recovery from repetitive, unhealthy habits, such as addictions. It is also effective with mental and emotional instabilities: depression, anxiety, and PTSD. CES produces a deep relaxation that increases suggestibility and allows new ideas and subconscious thoughts to surface.

Since its discovery in the late 1950s, micro-current stimulation has been used for pain relief. Early on, it was administered through a device that sent micro-current signals through the ears into the brain. The device was worn 23 hours each day for many weeks in an effort to treat heroin addiction, anxiety, depression, or insomnia.

Today, using the ThetaChamber℠ treatment can be accomplished much faster and more effectively by administrating micro-current stimulation while the brain is in the theta state. This method is done once or twice a day for 30 minutes. (While it takes much less time, treatment effectiveness is increased because of administering it while the brain is the most capable of receiving it.)

This FDA-approved treatment of micro-current stimulation uses subtle electrical impulses to affect the neural networks and neurochemistry of the brain, which encourages normal brain function. These electric signals are similar to those produced by the brain. The brain constantly sends and receives various signals back and forth from one region of the brain to another. Stress causes the electrical activity in your brain that regulates moods, emotions, sleep, and cognition not to function properly.

Once the brain has reached the theta state, the ThetaChamber℠ transmits gentle signals to the hypothalamus. These signals encourage the hypothalamus to start producing normal, healthy levels of serotonin, dopamine, and other neurotransmitters. This brings the brain, after a few applications, into more normal functionality. The results create new neural pathways, and the old, addicted, or imbalanced pathways atrophy.

Through decades of research and testing, doctors have been able to determine the precise frequencies, waveforms, amplitudes, and signal strengths needed to treat a variety of conditions. Anxiety, depression, and insomnia, as well as addiction to substances and stimuli: opiates, barbiturates, alcohol, nicotine, marijuana, cocaine, heroin, and pornography, can all be treated using precise frequencies. Each substance requires a different, specific, and precise setting for maximum effectiveness.

Research and a Meta-Analysis (data analysis from a number of independent studies on the same subject to determine overall trends) on depression treatment show CES treatment for depression is approximately two to six times more effective than antidepressant medication and has virtually no side effects.[15]

The use of CES for addiction was pioneered by Dr. "Meg" Margaret Patterson in the 1970s, beginning in Hong Kong. She understood that through electrical signals to the brain, she could introduce new wavelengths that would alter the production of serotonin, dopamine, and other feel-good chemicals, thus transforming destructive thoughts and emotions entrenched in the brain's biomagnetic field. By the late 70s, Dr. Patterson had perfected her techniques and was treating addiction with great success. She developed a following among professional musicians, including Pete Townshend, Eric Clapton, Keith Richards, and others who publicly claimed she saved their lives from drug addiction.[16][17]

It is a great source of joy to see lives and families restored as clients have overcome addictions that had seemed hopeless and previously "tried everything." A recent client expressed his relief and happiness at having no cravings after completing his treatment. He said, "This is amazing! Why aren't people lining up out the door to get helped here?"

---

[15] Guila MF and Kirsch DL, Cranial Electrotherapy Stimulation Review: A Safer Alternative to Psychopharmaceuticals in the Treatment of Depression, Journal of Neurotherapy, 2005, 9(2):7-24

[16] McAuliffe K., *Brain Tuner*, Omni, January 1983, 44-48, 115-120

[17] Patterson, M, *Hooked? NET: The New Approach to Drug Cure*, The Long Riders' Guild Press, 2007

Visual Light Pattern Stimulation

Visual Light Pattern Stimulation uses the same customized frequency to synchronize with the binaural beats to create a pattern of light that quickly induces the theta state. Computer-generated light patterns:

1) Quickly induce the theta state.
2) Open the brain to suggestion and entrainment.
3) Promote relaxing rhythms.

Light and sound sensory stimulation access the brain through the thalamus, which is directly connected to the cortex. Light, sound rhythms and patterns can easily influence cortical activity and affect neuronal activity when synchronized correctly.

The ThetaChamber℠ uses computer technology to generate and synchronize light, sound rhythms, and patterns together with micro-current signaling for a maximum positive effect. While the lights are white, many people report seeing colors and patterns through their closed eyes. That is the brain engaging with the light patterns.

Tanya's Story

Tanya had experienced a Traumatic Brain Injury (TBI) and was seeking treatment for PTSD, anxiety, inflammation, memory loss, and fatigue. After two weeks of treatment, she reported feeling less tired and lethargic, and her mood improved greatly. She began feeling more like herself and her energy had returned. Her program included using the ThetaChamber℠, Hyper-Cube hyperbaric oxygen therapy, rTMS, LED light therapy bed, and Brainspotting. She completed her program and now comes in for maintenance periodically as needed.

Norma's Story

Norma was in a car accident and had a Traumatic Brain Injury. Her distance vision would get blurry on occasion as a result. After the first session in the ThetaChamber℠, she remembers walking outside, and everything looked lighter and brighter; she could see distinct edges on the leaves of the trees. Her vision remained this way for about a week. A second treatment has resolved the problem with her vision. The ThetaChamber℠ did exactly what she hoped it would do. She said, "It balanced my brain super quick for me."

Lisandra's Story

Lisandra, 68, was struggling with memory. She was diagnosed with Cognitive Impairment a year prior to her seeking treatment at the Wellness Center and was told she was headed toward dementia. Three words into a sentence, her mind would go blank. She had trouble adding and subtracting simple numbers. The embarrassment caused her to stop talking at social events and instead just listen to others. Her family practice doctor took her off a medication he thought might be contributing and checked the vitamins and supplements she was taking. He ordered different diagnostic tests, a sleep study, etc. After meeting with a cognitive impairment specialist for a while, she was given computer exercises to do at home, which helped some.

This treatment was slow going. Then she found out about a program at the Theta Wellness Center in the city where she lived. Their approach was different from any other she had heard about, and used the ThetaChamber℠. She liked that the ThetaChamber℠ treatments were non-invasive. Lisandra was put on a program that included ThetaChamber℠, Hyper-Cube, and Hydrogen Therapy. In just one month, she had increased memory and was more able to do things she had done before the dementia advanced.

Patricia's Story

Patricia completed an intensive four-week program three times a week that focused on detox, and back and knee injury. She reported that since her program, she returned to her Orthopedist and was medically cleared to work out again! She began sleeping for longer periods and was feeling more rested. Generalized swelling and puffiness of her body decreased, and she reported, "Everything is improving."

Diane's Story

Diane, age 66, says, "The ThetaChamber℠ is an amazing modality!" She found that it has been extremely beneficial for depression, anxiety, and stress. Diane shared that she has also found that more stubborn issues like symptoms of PTSD have gradually diminished, and she has "felt" like her brain has been rewired back to a healthier, more balanced state.

Evelyn's Story

Evelyn, age 74, says the ThetaChamber℠ is a place where there is only "you with your thoughts, emotions, and feelings." She likes that it can be set for specific needs. Before using the ThetaChamber℠ she suffered from anxiety, feeling the difficulties of life crashing in. She reports that after using the ThetaChamber℠, she is more at peace with herself, relaxed, and refreshed to continue her life's journey.

Aiden's Story

Aiden, age 38, says the ThetaChamber℠ has been game-changing in managing depression, which he suffered his whole life. Since using the ThetaChamber℠, he has been able to better manage depressive cycles before they become a major obstacle to everyday functioning. He feels it has been a great contrast to the past, where it might take him months to regain that kind of balance.

Hyperbaric Oxygen Therapy

In a medically supervised hyperbaric oxygen chamber, the air pressure increases to three times higher than normal air pressure. Most people are familiar with using hyperbaric oxygen therapy to treat decompression sickness from scuba diving or altitude sickness. While it is very effective for both of those, there are many other beneficial applications.

Our low-pressure, ambient-air Hyperbaric Chamber is referred to as the Hyper-Cube. The Hyper-Cube is safer and more stable than other high-pressure oxygen chambers due to its low-pressure ambient air pressurization system.

How it Benefits the Body

Oxygen is so vital that being deprived of it for only a short time will lead to death. Oxygen fuels our cells, is necessary for constructing replacement cells for our bodies, and helps provide essential building blocks necessary for our survival. Every day about seven hundred billion cells in your body wear out and need to be replaced, which requires adequate oxygen for tissue regeneration. When tissue is injured, it requires even more oxygen to survive.

We live in a predominantly sedentary society; we sit, breathe shallowly, and don't move our bodies much, and the air we *do* breathe isn't pure. These factors leave many people without enough oxygen in their bodies to support the regular, daily functions of their internal and external organs (homeostasis). Hyperbaric oxygen therapy increases the amount of oxygen your blood can carry. Increased blood oxygen temporarily restores normal levels of blood gases and tissue function to promote healing and fight infection. Oxygen is a crucial part of our immune system and is used to help kill bacteria and fuel the cells that make up the body's defenses against viruses and other invaders.

Facts & Benefits of Low-Pressure Hyperbaric Therapy

Under normal circumstances, red blood cells transport oxygen throughout the body. With the Hyper-Cube, oxygen dissolves into the body's fluids, the plasma, central nervous system fluids, the lymphatic system, and the bones. During the dissolution, oxygen can be carried to areas of diminished or blocked circulation, helping the body support its healing process. This process dramatically enhances the body's ability for white blood cells to kill bacteria, reduce swelling, and allow new blood vessels to grow more rapidly in affected areas. The Hyper-Cube is simple, painless, and has a built-in Acoustic Light Wave and an oxygen concentrator. It comfortably seats two adults, but three have used it at the same time and seemed to have a good time. Some use their hour session to catch up on work, answer emails, or read. Many utilize the time to get very restful sleep.

When the body is injured by trauma, toxins, loss of blood flow, low oxygen, or other tissue damage, it causes the same secondary injury: an inflammatory reaction. Inflammation can be a healthy and normal body response. Inflammatory cells and cytokines (substances that stimulate more inflammatory cells) are your immune system's first responders. They trap bacteria, viruses, and toxic chemicals and start healing damaged tissue. The result is often pain, swelling, bruising, and redness. But inflammation also affects body systems you cannot see and can be a cause of many chronic diseases.[18]

The Hyper-Cube specifically treats the common secondary injury process responsible for most of the damage in all acute and chronic conditions. It also aids the acute inflammatory process and long-term products of the body's inflammatory reaction. Hyperbaric oxygen is one of the lowest-risk medical treatments available today. Conditions improved with hyperbaric oxygen used long-term include:

Fracture Healing	Bone Graft
Pre & Post Surgery Edema	Bacteroides Infection
Infection	Crush Injury
Cerebral Palsy	Autism
Acute Cerebral Edema	"Chemo" Brain
Emphysema	Post-Polio Syndrome
Intestinal Obstruction	Osteomyelitis
Soft Tissue Healing	Chronic Skin Ulcers
Stroke	Post Stroke Cortical
Multiple Sclerosis	Blindness
Lyme Disease	Symptomatic Dystrophy
Diabetic Ulcers & Neuritis	Skin Ulcers

---

[18] Cleveland Clinic, Inflammation: What Is It, Causes, Symptoms, & Treatment, https://my.clevelandclinic.org/health/symptoms/ 21660-inflammation#:~:text=Your%20immune%20system%20sends%20out, %2C%20swelling%2C%20bruising%20or%20redness.

Decubitus Ulcers	Gastric Ulcer
Peripheral Traumatic Ischemia	Angina
	Asthmas
Alzheimer's/Cerebral Vascular Disease	Traumatic Head & Spinal Cord Injury

Min's Story

Having been diagnosed with cancer, Min was advised to address problems with her lymphatic system and manage the stress that was too high. She wanted to help her body to capture the oxygen needed to promote healing in her body. In her first session with the Hyper-Cube, her coughing decreased. Before, when she went to bed, she would typically have a 2-minute bout of coughing before going to sleep. This particular time, when she went home, it was gone. Since using the hyperbaric chamber, she has not had coughing episodes before bed. She is looking forward to sharing the test results from her physician post-treatment. She is excited to share with others about the Theta Wellness Center. She says, "I'm glad that I've found it; it's a wonderful place to come."

Stan's Story

When he started treatment at the Theta Wellness Center, Stan, age 83, could not make it from his car to the center's front door without multiple stops to catch his breath. After treatments in the Hyper-Cube, he can now walk back and forth from his car to the clinic without stopping. Sessions in the ThetaChamber℠ and Hyper-Cube enabled him to improve his cognitive function and manage a huge contract job with sharper recall and improved math recall.

Amelia's Story

One of our youngest clients was three weeks old with fetal-related Hypoxia, showing limited mobility on the left side of her body. While there was no official diagnosis, her doctors hinted at Cerebral Palsy. She began using the Hyper-Cube chamber, lying on one of her parent's chests for one hour, five days a week, for several weeks. When she went to Stanford for her two-month checkup, there was no sign of the symptoms of CP or any other diagnoses given at birth.

Jacob's Story
A 39-year-old client, Jacob, sought treatment after being diagnosed with rectal cancer. Both pre-and post-surgery and throughout chemotherapy, he utilized the Hyper-Cube, Acoustic Light Wave, Hydrogen therapy, LED light bed, and Brainspotting. He reported that he felt better and healed faster.

LED Light Therapy Bed

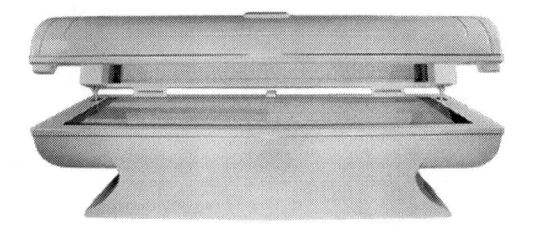

The LED Light Therapy Bed is simple to use, non-invasive, and has a long-standing history of therapeutic benefits. Although it may look like a tanning or light therapy bed, LED Light Bed Therapy is so much more. It is designed with 14,400 high-intensity red, blue and infrared LEDs positioned close to the skin for maximum effect. The LED lights activate Adenosine Triphosphate (ATP), stimulating white blood cells to repair damaged tissues, increasing collagen production, building elasticity in the skin, and aiding wound healing.

A contractor came in to work on the building where the clinic is located. Hunched over, he moved slowly in pain from a recently strained back with a pain level of ten out of ten. He lay in the light bed for a typical 20-minute session and reported no pain when he was done. Not only was he able to work with more ease, he then shared his experience with friends and family.

The LED Light Therapy Bed triggers the body's natural defenses, treating the source of pain rather than masking the symptoms. LED Light Therapy provides relief from pain and discomfort without harmful side effects. As our construction friend learned, specific wavelengths of light in the red and infrared spectrum can relieve many nerve, muscle, and joint conditions and benefit skin cells and other body tissues.

Red light therapy and infrared light therapy are used by professional athletes to promote healing with dramatic results and for those seeking cosmetic and anti-aging treatments. Red light therapy triggers the body's defenses and treats the sources of pain rather than masking symptoms. Red light therapy relieves pain and discomfort without any adverse effects.

The ATP production the LED Light Bed encourages utilizes the body's defenses and provides energy to drive many processes in living cells, such as muscle contraction, nerve impulse propagation, and chemical synthesis. An organic chemical found in all life forms, ATP is often referred to as the "molecular unit of currency" of energy transfer between cells.

ATP also helps to increase blood circulation, reducing swelling and inflammation. Increased blood circulation can benefit those with high blood pressure because good circulation allows the heart to do less work. It activates endorphins that provide soothing relief from chronic and acute pain. We learned of this machine from our sister, whose doctor referred her for LED Light Therapy after surgery. He knew the benefits it provided of shorter healing times for tissue.

Infrared light has the potential to trigger the production of endorphins, which are neurotransmitters that can reduce pain in the body. NASA research has shown that red light therapy and infrared light therapy can provide relief from:

High Blood Pressure	Joint Pain
Tissue and Nerve Damage	Arthritis
Chronic and Acute Pain	Acne
Decreasing Injury Healing Time	Rosacea
Backaches	Psoriasis
Neck Pain	Wrinkles
Muscle Pain	Bacterial Infection

The LED Light Bed has nine different programs utilizing the seven Nogier Frequencies. French physician Dr. Paul Nogier identified seven frequencies natural to our bodies. They became known as the Nogier Frequencies:

292 Hz – Cellular Vitality
Resonates with ectoderm (outermost tissue) that forms: skin, glands, nerves, eyes, ears, teeth, brain, and spinal cord, assists in wound healing, repair of the skin, nerve repair, reduces scar tissue, reduces inflammation, and reduces tumors.

584 Hz – Nutritional Metabolism
Resonates with endoderm (innermost tissue) that forms: lungs, bladder, urethra, the lining of the intestinal tract, liver, thyroid gland, thymus gland, auditory tube, gall bladder, pancreas, improves nutritional assimilation,

balances the parasympathetic nervous system and can alleviate allergy problems.

1,168 Hz – Movement
Resonates with mesoderm (middle tissue) that forms connective tissue: ligaments, tendons, cartilage, muscle and bone, heart, testes, cortex of the adrenal gland, blood, kidneys, lymph vessels, spleen, pain in muscles, skeletal or myofascial areas, and the ovaries.

2,336 Hz – Coordination
Coordinates the two sides of the brain and reduces stress.

4,672 Hz – Nerves
Pain, spinal cord, and skin disorders resonate with the spinal cord and the peripheral nervous system. The spinal cord carries the messages from the brain to all other parts of the body. The peripheral nervous system extends from the central nervous system. These nerves extend to the outermost areas of the body – to the organs, limbs, and skin.

73 Hz – Emotional Reactions
Balances hormones, muscle spasms, facial pain, headaches, depression, healing of non-healing bone fractures, balances thalamus, and hypothalamus – two major body control centers. Resonates with the subcortical or lower regions of the brain: speech, hormones balance, unconscious reactions/reflexes, memory, and improves circulation.

146 Hz – Intellectual Organization
Memory, psychological disorders, nervousness, and worry resonate with the brain's cerebral cortex: thinking, imagining, and creating: reduces inflammation and scar tissue on tendons and ligaments.

Jared's Story

Jared, age 10, was diagnosed with Eosinophilic Esophagitis (EoE). He was having a hard time swallowing and slowly stopped eating. Even though his doctor had him cut gluten from his diet, his symptoms progressed in severity. A biopsy several months later showed his white blood cells were too numerous to count. Food was getting stuck daily. Even after following his doctor's advice to eliminate gluten from his diet, the pain was so severe he could only eat about 200 calories a day. Dairy was eliminated, which resulted in some improvement, but eating remained painful.

One year later, he started using the LED red-light bed, noticing immediate improvement right away. He was able to eat normally. The pain resolved over time. His doctor ordered another biopsy. His white blood cell count decreased such that he no longer met the criteria for the diagnosis. He can focus better in school, play sports, and is more like himself again. He has been able to eliminate both the steroids and a medication that had intolerable effects.

Michael's Story

A couple of years ago, Michael, 76, was diagnosed with stage two prostate cancer. The recommended therapy was radioactive implants in his prostate, followed by three weeks of focused beam radiation. By the second week of radiation, he experienced: nausea, loss of appetite, diarrhea, fatigue, and more. The doctor told him his side effects could get worse before they got better.

He started a course of treatment with the Theta Wellness Center, including Hyperbaric Chamber sessions, breathing hydrogen, drinking hydrogenated water, and using a LED light bed. By the end of his 30-day program, he was feeling much better. When he went to the doctor for a follow-up exam, he asked Michael how he was feeling, and Michael replied, "Really good!" The doctor responded in surprise, "You are?"

At a follow-up physical, his family practice physician noted that his diabetic hemoglobin A1c decreased from 8 to 7.1. His doctor remarked, "I don't know what you are doing but keep doing it." In addition, Michael's PSA, a marker for prostate cancer, has remained at zero for almost two years now. Now, he is a firm believer in these treatments, continuing to use them periodically for health maintenance.

AO Scan Digital Analyzer

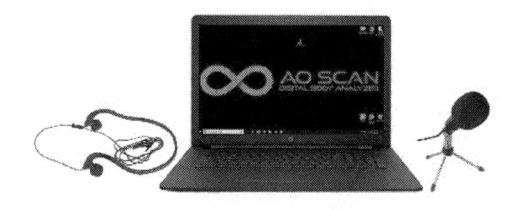

The AO Scan Digital Body Analyzer combines technology from Russia, Germany, Spain, Asia, and the USA. This technology is based on the science of Nikola Tesla, Dr. Royal Rife, Albert Einstein, and others who theorized that everything physical, fundamentally, has an energy frequency.

Biophysicists in Germany and Russia pioneered identifying specific frequencies in the human body. They compiled a database of more than 120,000 different blueprint frequencies representing homeostasis, that are the same for every person. (See Chapter Three.) Medical researchers in Germany found that the health of an organ, tissue, system, or cell structure within the body can be learned by passing frequencies through the body and measuring the current's resistance. It is similar to an electrocardiogram (ECG) or brain electroencephalogram (EEG). The brain is the body's CEO; everything reports to the brain in frequency output and response. The AO Scan takes those readings, analyzes them, computes them, and then sends them directly to the client.

The AO Scan Digital Body Analyzer is designed and built upon these proven technologies, utilizing today's technology to make the processes faster, more accurate, and unable to be intentionally or unintentionally influenced by the operator. The AO Scan Digital Body Analyzer completely and thoroughly scans the body's blueprint frequencies associated with 13 body systems and performs an optimizing analysis. The Vitals and Comprehensive scans generate a 50+ page data report sent directly to the client, highlighting body systems that need support. These systems include:

1. Circulation
2. Connective Tissue
3. Digestive
4. Endocrine
5. Lymphatic
6. Musculoskeletal
7. Nervous
8. Respiratory
9. Sensory Nervous
10. Integumentary (skin/Hair)

11. Urinary
12. Chromosomes
13. Human Cells & Mitochondria

Like other equipment at the Theta Wellness Center, the AO Scan Digital Body Analyzer is safe and non-invasive. It lists the detailed anatomy or components of each item it scans, offering an elegant yet simple method for measuring the energetic status of the entire body. The scan can project the energetic status out three to five years, providing detailed visual energetic status of the organs, systems, and tissue of the body and measuring electromagnetic signals and subtle bio-frequencies.

As stated, the working principles in the AO Scan Digital Body Analyzer system combine both the technologies of the past with the technologies of the present. Computers and computer hardware today can collect, process and analyze data at rates up to 1,000 times faster than equipment 10-20 years ago. The three main techniques the AO Scan System uses are:

1. Bio Resonance Recognition: The brain is the CEO of your body; every part of your body reports to the brain. In this technique, a specific signal is transmitted from the brain through a bone-conductor transducer headset into the Nuclear Localization Signal (NLS). This enables the brain to identify which part of the body is being scanned.

2. Bio Resonance Comparison: This process receives from the brain the resonating frequency of the part of the body that was selected and is then compared to the blueprint frequency of the selected organ, tissue, etc.

Then it compares the two frequencies, calculates how close they are to each other, and assigns a number from one to nine, with five being in perfect harmony and higher or lower than five indicating either stress or under activity.

3. Sympathetic Vibratory Physics: This process involves sending a sympathetic vibration back into the body to encourage the organ, tissue, etc., that is not within homeostatic range to move back towards the ideal range.

Inner Voice

The Inner Voice program helps harmonize your everyday life by improving concentration, creativity, and emotional intelligence. Your voice will always tell the truth, whether you want it to or not. When you talk or sing, you generate musical notes and chords that emotionally express to the listener characteristics and attributes of your personality, many of which are hidden in the subconscious mind. Your vocal cords carry your thoughts and emotions; no amount of masking your voice can change that fact.

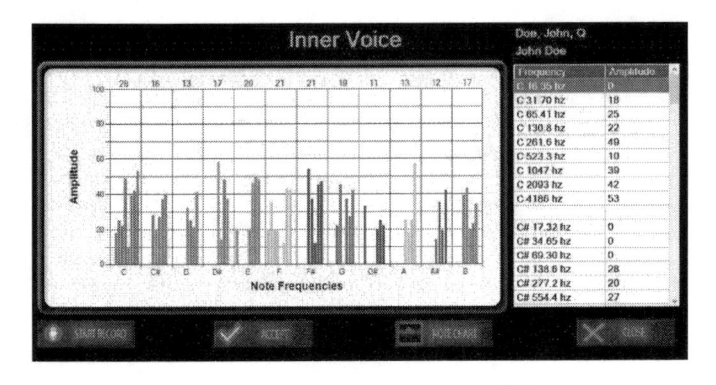

What we emotionally express through our voice profoundly affects our personal and business relationships and, in direct extension, our happiness and success. Our Inner Voice Scan utilizes the same technology as a lie detector test. You have a signature frequency that is unique to you. Inner Voice records 20 seconds of you speaking to identify your signature frequency, then isolates and analyzes imbalances in your emotional state (detected through your vocal cords).

Inner-Voice technology identifies three notes or octaves that are overactive and the primary octave being suppressed. Four 2-1/2-minute personalized MP3s are emailed to you (called balancing tones) to support your emotional and mental well-being. What you hear sounds like pleasant little tunes that provide all the balancing frequencies you need and diminish those in excess. A result is a powerful tool that helps rebalance your mental, emotional, and physical state of being.

Your emotions are important; your emotional state dramatically affects your ability to receive and hold onto healing. Long before the evolution of modern science, physicians and non-physicians agreed that a person's emotional state can affect how the body works. It has been estimated that 75-90 percent of all visits to primary care physicians are for stress-related problems.[19] The Center for Disease Control and Prevention (CDC) has stated that 85% of all diseases appear to have an emotional element. Studies indicate many chronic and even life-threatening diseases, including cancer, often begin with undealt-with emotions and stress from prior traumatic experiences.

---

[19] Paul J. Rosch, M.D., F.A.C.P, America's Leading Health Problem, USA Magazine, May 1991.

Do you want healing? It is a great idea to get emotionally balanced and healthy to support your healing journey.

Do you want the healing you have already received to endure? It is a great idea to get emotionally balanced and healthy.

AO Scan Inner Voice can help you.

April's Story
April, age 59, reported that after she had been listening to her tones for a couple of weeks, she began to feel more solid at her core, and things that really used to throw her off just didn't seem to bother her anymore.

Lauren's Story
Before having her Inner Voice scanned and listening to her tones, Lauren, Age 62, was feeling like a victim and having a hard time dealing with difficult things in her life. After listening to the tones for about 30 days, she no longer felt like a victim. She could stand up for herself and was better able to take care of things that would have caused her to struggle before.

Cherice's Story
Cherice, 58, reported having struggled with fear for years. After listening to balancing tones for two weeks, her husband asked her to go for a ride with him on his motorcycle. In the past, she declined out of fear, but this time she said, "Yes." She felt no fear, had a great time, and realized she would never have done that before.

Brady's Story
Brady, age 6, was challenged with being hyperactive with high emotion. After his Inner Voice, his parents noticed when playing his balancing tones, he would calm down or completely relax, often falling asleep.

Brandon's Story

Brandon, a 7-year-old client, was brought in for an AO Scan, had his Inner Voice recorded, and was sent his balancing tones. He had a strong history of physical outbursts and was extremely picky (and combative) about food. The mother said the food was always a fight. She reported that after only a couple of weeks of listening to his tones, he was less combative about food and generally doing better.

Vitals Scan

The AO Scan Digital Analyzer Vitals Scan is a non-invasive scan. By now, you know that each body part has a blueprint frequency, which is the frequency and vibration when in a balanced, normal state. Using a special bone-conductor (transducer) headset, the Vital Scan analyzes the frequencies of your blood biology. The scan helps you identify which areas are out of balance, then sends optimizing frequencies to assist the areas needing help. The scan generates reports before and after optimization in areas like toxicity, food sensitivities, heavy metals, nutritional analysis, and more.

The Vitals Scan quickly performs a complete scan of over 550 blueprint frequencies associated with each bodily function. It gives a concise snapshot of the frequencies produced by blood, organs, glands, and systems of the body in comparison to the blueprint frequencies. The results display the frequencies that are out of range with any blueprint. Reports include:

Blood report: educates about a range of blood measurements and displays frequency levels in and out of range. These include blood lipids, CBC, fatty acids, Omega-3, Omega-6, and fatty acid saturation.

Chakra report: Chakra derives from the Sanskrit word meaning wheel, circle, and cycle. This report displays each person's Chakra frequency levels and whether or not they are off balance.

Gastrointestinal report: educates about digestive function, inflammation/oxidation, and glucose homeostasis; displays the balances and imbalances of the gastrointestinal system frequencies.

Meridian report: displays the imbalances of the 12 Meridian lines: low (blue), normal (green), or high (red) functioning.

Nutritional report: displays normal or deficient measurements of macro- and micro-mineral, vitamin/co-enzyme, amino acid, and digestive acid/enzyme frequencies of the body.

Physical Functionality report: educates about frequency levels associated with a person's physical ability, bone and muscle condition, bone growth index, bone mineral density/disease, brain nerve, cardiovascular/cerebrovascular, collagen index, endocrine glands, eye health, hormones (mood, sex/sleep/stress), immune function, kidney function, liver and gall bladder function, lung function, reproductive body function, skin index, and thyroid function.

Toxicities report: educates about positive or negative frequency levels of toxicities, including environmental allergies/pollen, food allergies and sensitivities, bacteria, fungi, human toxins, molds, minerals, heavy metals, parasites, and viruses.

Comprehensive Scan

The Comprehensive Scan not only measures how well the body's systems are functioning but also projects the health status for three to five years. The result is a detailed visual health status of the body's organs, systems, and tissues. Fundamentally, the Comprehensive Scan is a functional test, not a medical diagnostic device. The scan determines functional vitality and can show early on the needed support and lifestyle changes required to restore function. It can pinpoint areas where help is needed, which standard tests may not show. It is a wellness tool (like a scale that measures weight, blood pressure cuff, glucose meter, or finger pulse oximeter) for people who want to take control of their health in today's confusing, complicated choices. It gives vital information to help you make better, informed decisions regarding any therapies, supplements, and changes you may want to consider.

The Comprehensive Scan gives detailed images similar to MRI, CT, or X-rays. It uses a bone-conductor transducer headset to scan over 130 organs, cells, bones, chromosomes, and systems in your body. It lists detailed components of each scanned item. It then produces a graphic report that identifies variances: when the response is low, vitality is lower; when high, the organ is under inflammatory stress. Frequency optimization picks up anything out of range. It generates balancing frequencies to help you balance your organs or systems to achieve complete balance. The report shows you the number of scores before and after balancing frequencies.

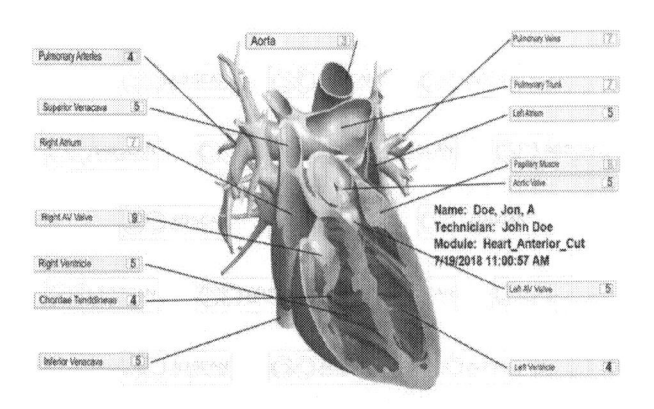

Reports may include:

Organs and Cells: informs about the cerebral cortex, brain sagittal, pancreas, prostate, liver, kidneys, lungs, blood, meninges, adrenal, cells, digestive system, skin, thyroid, gastrointestinal, chromosomes, basal ganglia, breasts, female sagittal, mitochondria, rectum, reproductive system, stomach, and urinary.

Veins: educates about the head, upper body, lower body, arms, and legs.

Skeletal: educates about the skull, teeth, spine, ribs, arms, legs, pelvis, hands, and feet.

Nerves: educates about the brain, head, upper body, lower body, legs, and arms.

Connective tissues: educates about the spine, eyes, hips, shoulders, elbows, feet, and knees.

Body Parts: educates about the muscles, head, arms, legs, hips, torso, neck, heart, ears, and lymphatic system.

Arteries: educates about the head, arms, upper body, lower body, and legs.

Repetitive Transcranial Magnetic Stimulation (rTMS)

Repetitive Transcranial Magnetic Stimulation (rTMS) uses magnetic fields to stimulate nerve cells in the brain. The stimulation supports the brain in creating and strengthening neurological pathways. rTMS is an innovative form of brain stimulation used to treat certain neurological disorders that have not improved through traditional approaches. Our software allows for personalized treatment sessions, which painlessly and safely deliver a magnetic pulse to activate different brain areas without the troubling side effects experienced by taking medication.

This process supports the brain in creating and strengthening neurological pathways. A typical session is 20-30 minutes. During an rTMS session, electromagnetic coils are placed against your scalp near your forehead. The electromagnet coil delivers magnetic pulses that stimulate your brain's nerve cells, improving neurologic activity in the affected areas. The procedure is safe and non-invasive.

rTMS redirects electric flow in the brain. Proper electric flow, in turn, generates proper chemical balance, which in turn results in the production of healthy amounts of "feel good" chemical messengers like serotonin and dopamine. This can result in the relief of even chronic symptoms seen in depression and other brain-related maladies.

A total of 289 studies on rTMS were published between 1990 and 2008, testing rTMS as a treatment tool for various neurological and psychiatric disorders, including migraines, strokes, Parkinson's disease, dystonia, tinnitus, depression, and auditory hallucinations. A Meta-Analysis in 2008 found rTMS effective for depression, with a greater effect than antidepressant medication.[20]

Transcranial Magnetic Stimulation was approved by the Food and Drug Administration (FDA) for the treatment of depression in 2008, expanded use for treating certain migraine headaches in 2013, and further expanded for the treatment of obsessive-compulsive disorder (OCD) in 2018.[21]

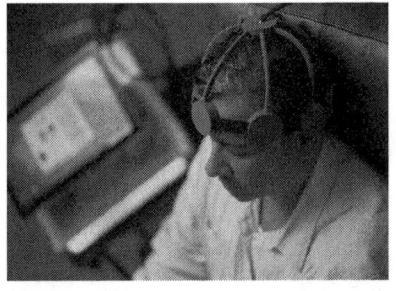

rTMS has been known to help treat the brain, ADD, ADHD, Depression, Alzheimer's, Parkinson's, chemical poisoning, addiction to chemical substances, brain fatigue, and traumatic brain injuries. Depending on the client's individual need, rTMS is

---

[20] Slotema CS et. Al. *Should We Expand the Toolbox of Psychiatric Treatment Methods to Include Repetitive Transcranial Magnetic Stimulation (rTMS)? A Meta-Analysis of the Efficacy of rTMS in Psychiatric Disorders.* J. Clin Psychiatry, 71:7, July 2010: 873-84

[21] *FDA permits marketing of Transcranial Magnetic Stimulation for treatment of obsessive-compulsive disorder*, FDA News Release, August 17, 2018

often used in conjunction with the ThetaChamber, LED light bed therapy, and sometimes the Hyperbaric chamber.

Ben's Story

Ben, age 23, had a history of autism spectrum disorder, diagnosed around age 17 years old. He had extreme social anxiety and could not be in a room with more than two or three people (even those he knew well) without having a panic attack or having to go down to the basement. He completed a 28-day program, including the ThetaChamber[SM], rTMS, and the Hyperbaric chamber. After the first two weeks, his grandparent had a dinner party for 16 people from out of town. They looked over and saw Ben sitting in the middle of the guests, immersed in conversation, introducing himself, and having a great time.

After the 28-day treatment, he went back home, where he lives with his mother. He is now one of the number-one salespeople for a well-known cellular phone company (in the Washington, Oregon, and Idaho regions). He loves his work and interacting with people so much that he works long hours, then volunteers on his days off. He has had such a drastic improvement in his social abilities that his mom says Theta gave her son back to her, but not the son she had known.

Marianne's Story

When 56-year-old Marianne came in, she had survived a massive Northern California fire. Her initial AO Scan showed frequencies indicating high levels of heavy metals, chemicals, mold, and fungus, and multiple allergies from breathing in the smoke. Suffering from PTSD, she also reported feeling physically toxic and emotionally challenged. After one week, she said she felt much better and that the previous night when she showered, "yellow water was coming out of my skin" and that she was generally not as tired and had more energy. After only a few weeks of protocol, she started feeling more settled and stable and reported that her skin was softer and more supple. As the detox program progressed, she and her husband noticed fewer emotional outbursts, greater mental clarity, and emotional stability.

5 HEALTH & WELLNESS THROUGH SCIENCE AND TECHNOLOGY

There are so many disorders and diseases we can support through our technology and modalities that it has been impossible to describe what we do in a one-minute "elevator speech." It has proven easier when people ask what we can do to, instead, to ask, "What do you need?" and go from there.

In addition to our main wellness centerpieces of equipment, we have additional science-based modalities that supplement the treatments we offer. Through these adjunct machines and modalities, we are able to serve our clients with highly individualized therapies. Here are some of the treatment options we offer:

Acoustic Light Wave (ALW)

Acoustic Light Wave uses a plasma tube antenna that emits a continuous, high-frequency wave through the air, similar to a radio tower. The radio transmitter excites a plasma gas formed within a glass tube. The energy emitted from the plasma tube antenna can be absorbed by an object when its resistance matches.

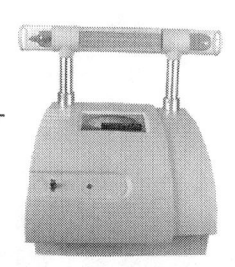

The resistance of the wave emitted from the plasma tube contrasts with microorganism frequencies (bacteria, viruses, etc.), disintegrating through membrane disruption in the body, according to Dr. Royal Rife. The ALW works to break down cell walls in pathogens and disease organisms. It is a drug-free, effective therapy with programmable capability for about 2,000 settings. Some protocols show benefits with one session.

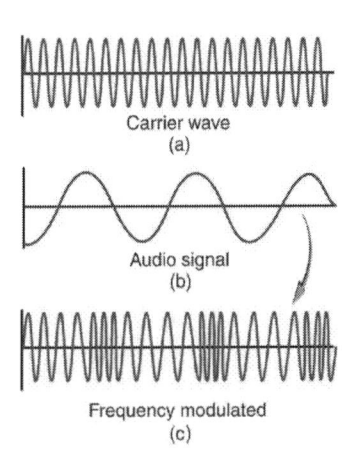

Carrier wave
(a)

Audio signal
(b)

Frequency modulated
(c)

The Acoustic Light Wave has been shown beneficial for use with:

Migraines	Symptoms of Common Cold
Sinus Issues	
Chronic Pain	Parasites
Bacteria	Bladder/Urogenital Discomfort
Virus	And more...

Corey's Story

Corey, age 39, says she is so glad that she found Theta Wellness Center because it changed her life! Out of work since 2011, she was able to go back to work after using the equipment. She suffered from insomnia (for five years), fatigue, and Lyme co-infections. She is now sleeping much better, and her co-infections have been cleared up. All this after following recommended protocols for only three months!

Dylan's Story

Dylan, age 10, had lingering effects from an infection that wasn't wholly clearing up, causing neurological challenges. He utilized the Acoustic Light Wave, with the hyperbaric to target the remnant of the infection. When he came to us, his brain was so over-firing that he could not calm down and rest. After four weeks of treatment, his parents noticed improvement. His dad reported that they attended several events and took a trip to the mall, where he did amazing. Previously the mall had been a difficult place for him to tolerate, making it impossible to take him there. His dad said, "On Sunday, he walked right by our side to the door and through the mall and was very regulated and enjoying himself. It was cool."

His dad recently updated us that Dylan is still doing exceptionally well. He is loving school and continues to be better at home as well. He reports that it has been wonderful for the entire family; they are having a lot of fun together. He credits Dylan's journey of improvement largely to the Theta Wellness Center and the help they received from the staff and equipment.

Hydrogen Therapy

Molecular Hydrogen protects extensively against oxidative stress, inflammation, and allergic reactions. Hydrogen is able to cross the blood-brain barrier and enter the mitochondria. Hydrogen is an anti-oxidant that never becomes a free radical in the body. Everybody can benefit from hydrogen therapy.

Hydrogen can be inhaled at low concentrations or infused into water and can protect cells from oxidative stress-related damage. As with all Theta Wellness Center technology, Hydrogen therapy is gentle, non-invasive, and safe.

Molecular Hydrogen is an innovative treatment for exercise-induced oxidative stress and sports injury. Increasing the oxygen levels in cells and tissues can reduce inflammation. When inflammation is reduced, clients report less pain and increased mental clarity and stamina. Used alone or paired with other therapies, it supercharges the body and ability to heal.

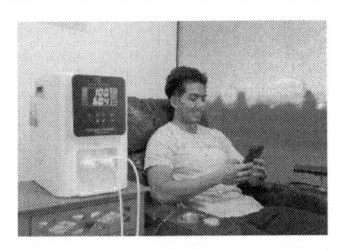

Hydrogen Therapy benefits may include but aren't limited to the following:

- Detoxification
- Ulcers and Sore Healing
- Minimizes Free-Radical Damage
- Lowered Cholesterol Levels
- Helps Flush Heavy Metals from the Body
- Improved Absorption of Supplements
- Improved Allergies and Asthma Conditions
- Better Blood Circulation
- Lowered Saturated Fat Levels
- Less Body Fatigue
- Faster Recovery from Diseases
- Improved Peripheral Circulation
- Improved Memory in the Elderly
- Boosted Brain Power
- Improved Bowel Function
- Improved Blood Glucose
- Reduction in Blood Pressure

Common testimonies using hydrogen include improved wound healing, reduction and elimination of swelling, improvement of sinus problems, improvement of headaches/migraines, increased energy, normalization of blood sugar, reduced need for insulin, feelings of refreshment, lightness in one's feet, increased alertness, stronger nails and hair, and improved joint flexibility.

Steve's Story
Steve, age 52, owns a gym and was previously a competitive bodybuilder. Over the years, he sustained numerous injuries with lingering pain. He reported that after having a single hydrogen treatment, he is pain-free for up to two days.

Thomas' Story
Thomas is a cardiac patient. He has had multiple procedures, such as bypasses and the placing of several stents. When he breathes Hydrogen for an hour, he feels stronger, with more energy. He says his brain seems sharper.

Presso-Therapy

Presso-Therapy helps the body by boosting blood circulation and lymphatic drainage, aiding in removing toxins and waste products.

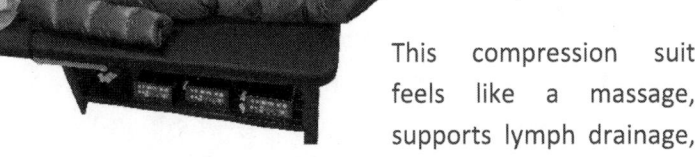

This compression suit feels like a massage, supports lymph drainage, improves blood circulation, and can reduce the appearance of cellulite.

Our Presso-Therapy Suit benefits may include but aren't limited to:

- Increased blood circulation
- Increased flow/drainage of the lymph nodes
- Improved ability to eliminate toxins
- Eliminated the appearance of cellulite
- Improved varicose veins
- Improved Thrombosis
- Improved ability to eliminate toxins

Jackie's Story

Jackie was seeking a program to help with uric acid building up in her joints and to help drain the lymphatic system. After three sessions of Presso-Therapy, she reported less pain in her joints. After several Presso Therapy sessions, she noted that her pelvic floor congestion was clearing up. She also experienced weight loss and a reduction of six inches of body fat.

Radio Frequency (RF) Detox

The RF Detox is a thermal shock-wave-depth conditioning instrument that circulates radio frequency (RF) vibration energy through the meridians of the feet to the whole body. Based on German micro-crystalline radio frequency vibration technology, our RF Detox treatments improve blood circulation deep within the cells of every body organ, raise the body's internal temperature to protect against disease, and support lymph health. Like any form of energy, RF Detox can produce heat.

An advantage of using radio frequency to heat tissues is that the lower frequency can safely penetrate to a deeper level.

According to Chinese medicine, creating heat can clear the meridians or energy points in the body, which clears blocked energy, improves immunity, and creates a healthy circulation of blood and energy from deep within the body. Raising the body's internal temperature by even one degree can increase immunity.

Raising the body's internal temperature can also create deep thermal resonance frequencies and accelerates blood circulation. Toxins and waste are broken down and sent to the liver, kidneys, and skin to be eliminated. Mucous, cholesterol, and fat, which can adhere to the arteries and vein walls, are dispersed and gradually can be eliminated by the body. Fresh oxygen and nutrients are circulated faster through the blood, detoxing the organs. Now cells and genes can start to be repaired and rejuvenated by the body. The RF Detox may help with some of the following:

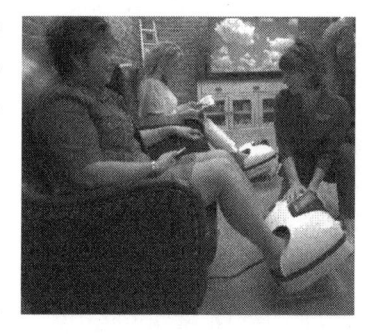

Hypertension	Hyperglycemia
Hyperlipidemia	Gout
Varicose veins	Backache
Muscle Atrophy	Joint pain
Weight loss	Skin Disease
Colds	Poor blood circulation
Neuropathy	And more...

Danni's Story
Danni, 38, did an RF Detox cleanse, which she absolutely loved! In the beginning, when she was detoxing really serious metals, she reported she could actually smell the burned metals coming

off of her. After a session and a half, her body no longer needed to detox from that anymore. She felt it all through her body.

Catherine's Story
Catherine, age 42, used the RF Detox for her lymphatic system. It had been so hard for her to sweat. She knew that because she was not sweating, she was not detoxing the body, so the RF Detox was giving her that boost. Catherine shared that in her sessions, she could actually feel the heat go up her legs and was breaking a sweat. She exclaimed, "It was phenomenal! It really helped me."

Nick's Story
Nick, age 65, had suffered from pain and neuropathy for years. He hadn't had a peaceful night's sleep for longer than he could remember. After using the RF Inner Cleanse, he had no pain in his legs. He went home and had a great night's sleep.

Warren's Story
Warren, age 74, said he had neuropathy in his feet for quite some time. They had been mostly numb with a constant tingling like pins and needles. After only a few sessions using the RF Inner Cleanse machine, he reported less tingling in his feet.

Vibration (Vibe) Plate

Vibration (Vibe) Plate Therapy uses whole-body vibration to modulate mood, metabolism, circulation, digestion, inflammation, muscle pain, joint pain, and nerve pain, improving overall energy. When you stand on a Vibe Plate, you can feel the vibration throughout your whole body; every cell throughout your body vibrates. This vibration causes a chain reaction, beginning with your muscle fibers involuntarily activating to tighten and relax at the same rate as the plate vibration. It also places gravity as your muscles hold your weight, which leads to beneficial results.

The benefit of ten minutes on a Vibe Plate has been compared to one hour of weight lifting; it increases muscle strength, flexibility, bone density, balance, coordination, and weight loss (without the heavy lifting.)

Exercise is an important factor in brain health, as it stimulates neural cell growth and strength. The Vibe Plate creates neurological stimulation as your neurons send signals (20-50 per second) to your brain. Just as your body is growing stronger, your brain and neurological system do too. Some of the Immediate, beneficial side effects include the production of the neurotransmitters serotonin and norepinephrine, positively affecting your mood and energy levels.[22]

A recent New York Times magazine article states, "For more than a decade, neuroscientists and physiologists have been gathering evidence of the beneficial relationship between exercise and brainpower. It isn't a relationship; it is *the* relationship. Exercise, the latest neuroscience suggests, does more to bolster thinking than thinking does."[23] While professional athletes have been using vibration for years to enhance performance, this therapy benefits anyone interested in improving their health.

---

[22] Becky Chambers, *Homeopathy Plus Whole Body Vibration, Combining Two Energy Medicines Ignites Healing*, Quartet Books, Charlottesville, VA, 2016
[23] Gretchen Reynolds, Jogging Your Brain, New York Times Magazine, April 2012, 46.

Whole-body vibration has many benefits. You can sit, stand, stretch, and move on the Vibe Plate, enhancing your strength, balancing hormones, increasing lymphatic drainage, increasing bone mass, improving circulation and balance, enhancing blood flow, reducing muscle soreness after exercise, decreasing stress (cortisol) hormones, as well as reducing inflammation levels.

Treatments are ten minutes and can be helpful for the circulatory and lymphatic system body moving for maximum benefit when using other modalities. We use it in our Jump Start Weight Loss Program.

James' Story
James, age 42, said, "I have never experienced anything like this. I feel great – this is healing in new ways."

Brainspotting[24] Trauma Therapy

Brainspotting (a proprietary term and trauma therapy created and named by David Grand, Ph.D.) is a powerful, focused treatment method that works by identifying, processing, and releasing emotional and body pain, trauma, dissociation, and challenging symptoms. When someone experiences trauma, the traumatic feelings often get "locked" within the body. A brain spot is actually a physiological substation holding an emotional experience in memory form. Different from talk therapy, Brainspotting functions as a neurobiological tool to support the clinical healing relationship.

Brainspotting is an innovative therapy that combines aspects of EMDR, mindfulness, and brain-body-based therapies. Developed

---

[24] David Grand, *Brainspotting: The Revolutionary New Therapy for Rapid and Effective Change*, Sounds Good Books, April 2013

by David Grand through his work with first responders and survivors of 9/11, it accesses trauma trapped in the subcortical brain (the area of the brain responsible for motion, consciousness, emotions, and learning). Brainspotting is a technique that helps people process trauma and resolve it.

Trauma can be caused by any surprising or terrible physical or emotional event (real or imagined) in which a person experiences being overwhelmed, helpless, or trapped. It is estimated that half of Americans will go through a traumatic event at least once in their lives. Tragedy, chronic pain, serious illness, medical interventions, societal turmoil, and environmental threats/disasters all add to stored trauma.

Trauma that is stored in the body does not release on its own.[25] The result is seen in rising requests for medical care linked to stress and trauma of the body. Unlike traditional talk therapy, Brainspotting does not rely on retelling or living the trauma again but focuses on releasing the reservoir of maladaptive feelings trapped in the body. It is based on the premise that where you look determines what you feel.

A brain spot is the eye position related to an energetic or emotional activation of a traumatic (emotionally charged) issue within the brain. Such memories are usually held beyond the pre-frontal cortex (which handles linear, logical, and sequential thinking) in the amygdala, the hippocampus, which encodes memory.

Brainspotting works with the deep brain and the body through its direct access to the autonomic and limbic systems within the

---

[25] Bessel A. van der Kolk, MD, *The Body Keeps Score: Brain, Mind, and Body in the Healing of Trauma*, Penguin Books, 2014

body's central nervous system. In sessions, the client is seen as an expert on themselves; therefore, the therapist operates in a supporting role. You can talk as much or little as you would like during the session: you can process internally or verbally share as things come up. Brainspotting offers dignity and privacy to those who have experienced trauma but have difficulty talking about it. It assists with releasing neurophysiological sources of emotional and body pain, trauma, and other challenging symptoms.

Brainspotting can be an effective and efficient treatment for:
- Anxiety
- Attachment Issues
- Physical and Emotional Trauma
- Stress and Trauma-Related Medical Illness
- Recovery from Injury and Accident Trauma
- Addictions
- Anger and Rage Problems
- Post-Traumatic Stress Disorder
- Chronic Pain
- Anxiety and Panic
- Major Depressive Disorder
- And more...

Nita's Story
Nita had a session of Brainspotting and reported that it was "PHENOMENAL!" She said it only took one session and she felt the weight off her shoulders. She had a knot in her neck for two months that would not go away. After that session, her muscles were less tense, and she realized the knot in her neck was gone. She was extremely pleased.

Alex's Story

Alex, 28 years old, reported how much lighter and better she felt after one session. Her favorite part was not having to talk about the details of events and memories but still getting great relief.

Doug's Story

After years of anxiety, sadness, fear, and feeling like a victim because of childhood abuse, Doug, 52, said after Brainspotting, he felt like a different person. It was as if a huge weight had been lifted from his neck, shoulders, and stomach. He had often felt controlled by his partner. After Brainspotting, he explained that he now saw his spouse in a completely different light; he realized he had been seeing their interactions through a victim mentality. Doug is excited about his emotional freedom and the changes he is already seeing in his marriage.

Kyle's Story

Kyle, 38, didn't know what to expect with Brainspotting – it was part of a treatment plan designed for him by the Theta team. He came to the Theta Wellness Center after treatment for cancer to help him lessen the side effects of chemotherapy and radiation. He experienced great results from his program; he just wasn't sure about "Brainspotting." Once he got started, he realized he was holding on to extreme fear of not being around to see his children grow up, play sports, and, perhaps, one day get married or have children. He was able to release those fears as well as the trauma he experienced through his cancer diagnosis and treatment. After, he felt so good that he asked if he could hug everyone in the center.

Gayle's Story

Gayle, 72, came in for Brainspotting because she was feeling panicked about having her whole extended family over for Thanksgiving at her house. Some of the family members were very critical, others insisted on their way, several didn't contribute or help, and she knew it would all lead to more work for her. In her Brainspotting session, she realized the feelings about being criticized for not doing things perfectly and resentment for others putting their high expectations on her went way back. As her body was able to release the trauma she had been storing, she began to relax and no longer felt anxious about her houseguests. She also realized she was empowered to ask for (and expect) help. Gayle later reported that she made it through the long Thanksgiving weekend with minimal stress.

> "When all you know is fight or flight,
> red flags and butterflies all feel the same."
> -Cindy Cherie, Australian Poet

6 EMOTIONAL & MENTAL HEALTH

Taking care of your emotional and mental health is not a frivolous option, as some people have historically thought. Emotional and mental health are major concerns in schools, businesses, the private and public sectors, relationships, families, and the community at large. The urgency can be seen in directives and funding increases.

In 2022, America's Department of Health and Human Services (HHS) made over a billion dollars available in grant funding for community mental health services and suicide prevention programs for children and young adults. That same year, billions were invested in California's mental health system to boost coverage options and public awareness so children and youth could be routinely screened, supported, and served.

Between 2016 and 2020, the number of children, ages 3-17 years, diagnosed with anxiety grew by almost a third; those with depression grew by over 25%. Further, in 2020, suicide was the leading cause of death for young people aged 10-14 and 25-34, according to the HHS Centers for Disease Control (CDC).

Employee mental well-being programs have been instituted, and insurance funds have been made available for employees and employers straining under social, business, and government stressors. Employers are getting wise to the fact that when their employees' emotions are balanced, it can reduce emotional stress, give relief for anxiety, enable better focus, increase creativity, and foster the ability for better work-life balance.

At Theta Wellness Center, we work with the brain to help the body produce the feel-good hormones and neurotransmitters necessary for better mental health. We focus on getting both the body and brain back into a healthy state. If the brain-body foundation isn't strong, it is difficult to sustain mental healing over time. We have protocols that utilize brain science to give clients an advantage to better health.

Addiction/Substance Abuse

According to the Substance Abuse and Mental Health Services Administration (SAMHSA), 9 out of 10 people who need substance abuse treatment do not get it. According to the National Institutes on Drug Abuse (NIDA), drug-related deaths have more than doubled since the early 1980s. More deaths, illnesses, and disabilities from substance abuse exist than from any other preventable health condition. Today, one in four deaths is attributable to alcohol, tobacco, or illicit drug use.

When confronted with injury, illness, and difficulties in life, it is not uncommon for people to turn to alcohol or drugs to cope with and mask daily stress. Afflictions come in many forms that change brain circuitry. Addiction isn't always obvious; it can affect all generations and socioeconomic people groups and often involves a substance or activity that is common and/or legal. Vulnerability can begin with the first use. We have yet to run across anyone who set out on a journey to become an addict.

Relapse rates for addictive diseases usually are typically 50% to 90%. These rates vary by definition of relapse, the severity of addiction, addictive drug, length of treatment, elapsed time from treatment discharge to assessment, as well as other factors.[26]

For example, under traditional care, one year after stopping opiates (a substance found in certain pain medications and illegal drugs like heroin), there is an 85% chance of relapse. According to the NIDA, addiction changes brain circuitry, making it hard to "apply the brakes" to detrimental behaviors. In the non-addicted brain, control mechanisms constantly assess the value of stimuli and the appropriateness of the planned response. Inhibiting control is then applied as needed. The addicted brain control circuit becomes impaired because of drug use, so it loses much of its inhibiting power over the circuits that drive responses to stimuli deemed important. In other words, altered brain chemistry inhibits your ability to limit or stop future use of something that will cause further altered brain chemistry.

Each addiction has its own unique set of challenges. To overcome smoking, you must deal with the actual addiction to the 600-plus chemicals in a cigarette (American Lung Association), the neurological habit, and the hand-to-mouth behavior.

Heroin, known to be one of the most dangerous and addictive substances known to mankind, is currently so easy to find and cheap to get that is an epidemic among unhoused communities.

---

[26] Winfred Wu, MD, Amy J Khan, MD, MPH, *Adolescent Illicit Drug Use: Understanding and Addressing the Problem*, American College of Preventive Medicine, Medscape Pubic Health and Prevention 2005;3(2)

You may be aware of the widespread opiate crisis that cuts across economic and societal barriers and has placed a major resource strain on the medical community. Many think that addiction to cocaine is much harder to beat than sugar, but did you know that sugar is only one molecule away from cocaine?

Pornography is as hard to kick as heroin. Dr. Donald L. Hilton, Jr., Clinical Associate Professor, University of Texas Health Sciences Center at San Antonio, states that pornography has the ability to re-program the brain structurally, neurochemically, and metabolically.

On August 15, 2011, the American Society of Addiction Medicine issued the following public statement defining all addictions (including sexual behavior addiction) in terms of brain changes. "Addiction is a primary, chronic disease of brain reward, motivation, memory, and related circuitry." That explains the exponentially increasing cases of video gaming disorder and internet use addiction.

Any addiction treatment that fails to normalize brain chemistry has little chance of long-term success. Theta Wellness Center's addiction program is faster and more effective than other addiction programs that do not use ThetaChamber[SM] technology. We support clients in overcoming the following addictions: alcohol, drugs, gaming, pornography, sugar, and more.

Our addiction protocol includes:

ThetaChamber[SM]: synchronizes neural pathways, reduces stress hormones, and resets brainwaves.

LED Light Bed: reduces emotional stress, activates endorphins, and balances the thalamus and hypothalamus.

AO Scan Digital Body Analyzer: includes comprehensive full body scan, vitals report, and supports balanced emotions with optimizing tones.

rTMS: increases serotonin and dopamine, synchronizes neural pathways, and stimulates brain cells.

Brainspotting therapy is often integrated based on personal needs.

Lydia's Story

For years, Lydia, age 43, had struggled with a sugar addiction - she had no "stop" button. Since completing the Jump Start program, she said she literally had no sugar cravings. She added, "The other day, I was feeling hungry and realized I was wanting celery and carrots. That has never happened before."

Richard's Story

Richard came to Theta Wellness Center to address tobacco and alcohol addiction. On his first day, he had a severe hangover and was skeptical about how the ThetaChamber℠ would work for him. After his first session, he decided to smoke a cigarette. He felt immediately nauseous and turned off by the taste and smell. Richard had been smoking for many years but had to put it down after one drag. He continued with his ThetaChamber℠ treatments every day for ten days and testifies that he has not desired another drink since the first treatment. He says he will continue coming to Theta Wellness Center once a week to maintain his progress because it has improved the quality of his life and helped him kick his bad habits.

David's Story

David, age 44, recently had a heart attack while on methamphetamines and came to us for treatment for addiction.

He had been using drugs regularly since he was around 19 years old. While his friends had gone on to use cocaine and heroin, he didn't like either. He had been using Fentanyl for about six months but knew he was playing with death. He had previously gone through a 12-Step program and several inpatient and outpatient programs. He didn't like the group sessions and rarely participated in the discussions unless called upon. He felt the programs he tried were largely unsuccessful because nothing changed inside him and because he thought addicts helping addicts doesn't work. He was hopeful the Theta Way would work because of the science. He believed our brains and bodies can change and be healed. Having a heart attack caused him to look for something different.

At the end of his program, he felt physically changed. The cravings went away and he was confident he could continue moving forward and would not use it again. He felt so good he wondered why people aren't lined up out the door to get in for treatment. He left as a satisfied client, armed with a new skill set and tools to maintain freedom.

Todd's Story

Todd, age 30, had been addicted to heroin since age 15. He came into the Theta Wellness Center to deal with withdrawal and his addiction. He had been unable to sustain sobriety after several other programs and now suffered from mental health challenges, including anxiety, severe depression, and anger, all brought on by his heroin addiction. After detoxing, he completed a 21-day addiction protocol. In the first two weeks of the program, he had high anxiety and nausea. After that, he felt calmer and more in control of his life. To date, Todd has sustained clean and sober living. He says that Theta Wellness

Center is the best and most efficient program for him because it dealt with the brain and not just his behavior.

Sandy's Story

Sandy, 47, had surgery for a herniated disk, which led to chronic neck pain. As a result, she was prescribed and became addicted to opiates for five years. Her husband left and divorced her because he could no longer deal with her addiction. After detoxing, she started a 21-day addiction program. By the last day, she had developed tools to work on relieving pain using healthy methods and, in the past seven years, has never gone back to using opiates. Sandy is now remarried and is grateful for her new life made possible by kicking her opioid addiction at the Theta Wellness Center.

Anthony's Story

Anthony, age 48, had unsuccessful back surgery at age 27, which left him with severe and chronic pain. Later, he also experienced trauma from a car accident and emotional family circumstances about this time. His doctor originally prescribed oxycodone for the pain, but the prescription eventually ran out. Anthony had no problem getting more pills from other sources. Initially, the oxycodone provided a sense of euphoria and helped him deal with life. Over time, he increased from 1-10 pills a day to 80 a day.

After asking for help, Anthony was admitted to a state-funded treatment center. He lasted two weeks, then climbed out the window and left. Because money had not been an issue for him, he had since gone through seven of the most expensive drug rehabilitation centers and programs in the U.S. Some cost up to $95K for one month. When he was in the centers, he learned ways to feed addiction, such as: where to get cocaine, new drugs to try, how to score them, and how to get drugs while in rehab. He spent hundreds of thousands of dollars in efforts to get clean prior to going through the Theta Way technology. Anthony says the biggest difference is his cravings are now gone. He is now able to move forward in his life.

Depression

Depression manifests differently in different people. It can affect how a person thinks and feels about themselves and how they handle daily activities, such as sleep, eating, physical aches and pain, fatigue, and feelings of hopelessness. Depression is commonly treated with psychotherapy and antidepressants, which can impair the ability to manage day-to-day activities.

Depressive Disorders include the following three categories. The first, Major Depression, interferes with the ability to eat, sleep, work, study, or enjoy once-pleasurable activities. It may occur once or recur frequently. Second, Dysthymia is long-term, with chronic symptoms. It is not disabling but doesn't feel good. Those with dysthymia may experience episodic major depression on top of dysthymia. Third, Bipolar Disorder includes cyclic mood changes between severe highs (mania) and severe lows (major depression). It may be dramatic or gradual. Depressive Disorders affect almost 20% of U.S. adults and over 10% of adolescents. One in four women and one in ten men will suffer from depression at some point in their lifetime.

Depression causes more absenteeism than almost any other physical disorder, costing employers more than $51 billion per year in lost productivity. This reflects in high medical and pharmaceutical bills. The total spent on antidepressants/antipsychotics in 2018 was over $28 billion[27]. Depression destroys productivity, relationships, and quality of life. The result: suicide is now the fourth leading cause of death among U.S. adults.

Though counseling has historically been used for depression, the increasing availability of pharmaceuticals seems to have overshadowed counseling as a treatment choice. Antidepressants (and anti-psychotics) are now the most-prescribed class of drugs in the U.S. However, recent studies increasingly show antidepressants are no better than placebos and carry serious risks, such as increased risk of suicide, particularly in young people.

Nevertheless, depression "treatment" remains a significant and lucrative market, primarily because antidepressant drugs are commonly prescribed but rarely de-prescribed. The New York Times reported that before Covid, the number of Americans taking an antidepressant was one in eight Americans.[28] By many accounts, that number has increased since 2020. Because altered brain chemistry is the root of the problem, any treatment that fails to normalize brain chemistry has little chance of long-term success. We use a neurological approach to correct chemical imbalances in the brain. Brain therapy has been shown to be an effective treatment option.

Protocols for Depression:

> **ThetaChamber℠**: synchronizes neural pathways, reduces stress hormones, and resets brainwaves.
>
> **LED Light Bed**: reduces emotional stress, activates endorphins, and balances the thalamus and hypothalamus.

---

[27] https://www.ahrq.gov/data/visualizations/prescription-antidepressants.html, Agency for Healthcare Research and Quality
[28] https://www.nytimes.com/2022/11/08/well/mind/antidepressants-effects-alternatives.html

AO Scan Digital Body Analyzer: includes comprehensive full body scan, vitals report, and supports balanced emotions with optimizing tones.

rTMS: increases serotonin and dopamine, synchronizes neural pathways, and stimulates brain cells.

Brainspotting therapy is often integrated, as needed.

Janie's Story

Janie, age 49, had dealt with severe depression and anxiety for most of her life. She was intrigued by Theta Wellness Center and how different we are from what she had already tried. After completing treatment for a month, she reported her results were nothing short of a miraculous transformation! Her anxiety decreased immensely, hormones were more regulated, she no longer had insomnia issues, and was able to come off medications. She also worked with our nutritional coach, who gave her tools to take care of herself, which she says helped exponentially. She reported that she can't say enough about Theta Wellness Center and the wonderful staff.

Post-Traumatic Stress Disorder (PTSD)

PTSD is a severe anxiety disorder affecting people who have survived severe trauma. PTSD is a complex condition characterized by recurrent, intrusive memories, distressing dreams, flashbacks, and/or severe anxiety about a terrifying event experienced or witnessed. As with other stress-related disorders, it involves a chemical imbalance in the reward circuit of the brain. PTSD manifests itself in a wide variety of symptoms and effects. For any treatment to be effective, it must correct the imbalances in the brain associated with PTSD.

Though PTSD is most common among combat veterans, it also affects accident and assault victims, first responders, and others who suffer traumas. People with PTSD have among the highest rates of healthcare service use. Presenting with a range of symptoms which may be overlooked or undiagnosed as having resulted from past trauma. According to the National Institutes of Mental Health (NIMH), PTSD can cause many symptoms.

These symptoms are grouped into three categories:

1. **Re-experiencing symptoms** can include flashbacks or reliving the trauma repeatedly, including physical symptoms like a racing heart, sweating, bad dreams, and frightening thoughts. They can cause problems in a person's everyday routine. They can start from the person's thoughts and feelings. Words, objects, or situations that are reminders of the event can also trigger re-experience.

2. **Avoidance symptoms** may include: staying away from places, events, or objects that are reminders of the experience; feeling emotionally numb; feeling intense guilt, depression, or worry; losing interest in activities that were enjoyable in the past; and having trouble remembering the dangerous event.

Things that remind a person of the traumatic event can trigger avoidance symptoms. These symptoms may cause a person to change their personal routine. For example, after a bad car accident, a person who usually drives may avoid driving or riding in a car.

3. **Hyperarousal symptoms** may include: being easily startled, tense, or "on edge," having difficulty sleeping or having angry outbursts. Hyperarousal symptoms are

usually constant instead of being triggered by things that remind one of the traumatic events.

They can make the person feel stressed and angry. These symptoms may make it hard to do daily tasks, such as sleeping, eating, or concentrating.

According to HealMyPTSD.com, among people who are victims of a severely traumatic experience, 60-80% will develop PTSD. Almost 50% of all mental health outpatients have PTSD, and an estimated 8% of Americans, or 31.3 million people, have PTSD at any given time. As with our other treatment plans, our neurological approach is tailored to each individual and their specific needs. We incorporate some of the following equipment into our programs:

ThetaChamber[SM]: synchronizes neural pathways, reduces stress hormones, and resets brainwaves.

LED Light Bed: reduces emotional stress, activates endorphins, and balances the thalamus and hypothalamus.

AO Scan Digital Body Analyzer: includes comprehensive full body scan, vitals report, and supports balanced emotions with optimizing tones.

rTMS: increases serotonin and dopamine, synchronizes neural pathways, and stimulates brain cells.

Brainspotting therapy is often integrated, as needed.

Dirk's Story
Dirk, age 52, shared that he had experienced many traumas in his life: childhood abuse, the trauma of pulling two teenagers from a burning car, and the atrocities of war, including having to

pick up body parts off the road. By the time he was discharged from the military, he was diagnosed as 70% disabled because of PTSD. Because of this high percentage of disability, he was able to quickly go into the Veteran's Administration program for treatment with PTSD (ahead of the usual two-year waiting list). Going to weekly group appointments where he talked about those events made him actually worse.

After being in the program for about three years, feeling re-traumatized every week by the group sessions, he found out about the ThetaChamber℠. After 28 days of using the ThetaChamber℠ every day, he believed he no longer had PTSD. Dirk did due diligence and went back to the V.A. for verification. He was re-diagnosed as 30% disabled but knew they just did not know how to justify his healing. He says he can now function very well in daily life. Because of his own positive healing experience, he is now committed to helping other veterans get help for the crippling mental and emotional stress that can come with PTSD.

Stress & Anxiety

Stress is a response to a threat or short-term experience that can manifest itself in a number of mental and physical symptoms. Anxiety is a reaction to stressful life situations which can create constant fear and worry and even become overwhelming and disabling. Stress and Anxiety disorders involve a chemical imbalance in the reward circuit of the brain.

Anxiety Disorders are the most common mental illness in the U.S., affecting almost 20% of adults and 25% of adolescents. Anxiety disorders include the following:

- Generalized Anxiety Disorder
- Panic Disorder
- Post-Traumatic Stress Disorder
- Obsessive-Compulsive Disorder Phobias

Anxiety disorders cost the United States more than $42 billion a year, almost one-third of the $148 billion total mental health bill for the U.S. (1999 numbers)[29]. Half of these costs are associated with repeated healthcare services because people with anxiety disorders seek relief from symptoms that mimic physical illnesses.

People with an anxiety disorder are three-to-five times more likely to go to the doctor and six times more likely to be hospitalized for psychiatric disorders than non-sufferers. Women are twice as likely to be afflicted as men, and anxiety disorders are very likely to co-exist with other disorders.

Various types of counseling have traditionally been used to address and treat anxiety disorders. However, the increasing availability of anti-anxiety drugs and staffing shortages within the mental health community have repositioned counseling: it is often combined with medication and is not always the first step of effective treatment. Interestingly, the largest increase in the use of anti-anxiety medications in the past ten years has been among teenagers. The rise in anti-anxiety prescriptions has also increased drug abuse. According to NBC New York, a surge in prescription drug abuse involving Xanax and similar anti-anxiety pills has prompted some doctors in the U.S. to rethink the frequency with which they dole out the prescription.

---

[29] PE Greenberg et.al, *The economic burden of anxieties in the 1990s*, https://pubmed.ncbi.nlm.nih.gov/10453795 DOI: 10.4088/jcp.v60n0702 1999 Jul;60(7):427-35.

Between 2004 and 2009, New York City emergency room visits involving Xanax and other anti-anxiety prescription drugs, known as benzodiazepines, increased by more than 50 percent. That's up from 38 out of 100,000 New Yorkers in 2004 to 59 out of 100,000 New Yorkers. Data from the New York City Department of Health also show benzodiazepines were tied to more than 30 percent of all the city's overdose deaths in 2009 or 3.3 out of 10. Nearly all of those overdoses involved multiple drugs, of which benzodiazepine was just one.

We offer a drug-free, non-invasive technology for better brain health that is safe and effective in a protocol that includes:

ThetaChamber℠: synchronizes neural pathways, reduces stress hormones, and resets brainwaves.

LED Light Bed: reduces emotional stress, activates endorphins, and balances the thalamus and hypothalamus.

AO Scan Digital Body Analyzer: includes comprehensive full body scan, vitals report, and supports balanced emotions with optimizing tones.

rTMS: increases serotonin and dopamine, synchronizes neural pathways, and stimulates brain cells.

Brainspotting therapy is often integrated, as needed.

Laura's Story

Laura, age 34, came to Theta Wellness in an attempt to calm her anxiety and stress. She described the ThetaChamber℠ as a unique experience. She was in the pod for 30 minutes, and it felt like a lucid dream. When her time was up and the pod had stopped spinning, she sat up and could not stop smiling. She exclaimed that she was as relaxed as she would have been after 10 hours of sleep and felt extremely euphoric. She felt substantially more relaxed than after an hour-long massage.

Her drive home was filled with traffic and other irritants, but she was still very relaxed. Laura fell asleep very early that night, an interesting and unexpected effect for someone who frequently experienced insomnia. That night, she slept through the night, having the most wonderful dreams. The next morning, she was still extremely calm and content down to the core. Laura *highly* recommends Theta Wellness and the ThetaChamber℠.

Meaghan's Story
Meaghan went to Theta Wellness Center eight years ago. She had been dealing with fibromyalgia, gut issues (including parasites), stress, anxiety, and PTSD. In her quest for better health, she had previously sought and utilized some use of frequency for health support and was familiar with its healing qualities. While Meaghan had experienced some healing, she was ready to take it to the next level.

One day, she had a conversation with her sister about this, and her sister said, "I think I found what you are looking for. I took my son to the inventor who created the ThetaChamber℠ bed for a neurological reset. He was treated on a 28-day program for stress and anxiety." Meaghan thought, "Wow! I want to meet him too. Maybe he can do something for me!"

She set up an appointment and drove 300 miles to Theta Wellness Center. She was really excited. During her consultation, Loran Swensen said, "I think I know what you need, and I am going to run an AO Scan on you." He went over the scan results with her. It showed everything from her past history; she was blown away! She wondered how a machine could know what was going on in her body and with her emotions: that she had crushed her foot bones, her shoulder was out of place, she had a history of shingles and more. Using that information, Loran was able to pinpoint what she needed.

Meaghan made a commitment to ten weekly sessions. Each week at a designated time, Loran called and, using a remote device, performed a 45-minute scan. After, she was so energized she could take a 30-minute hike (something that had been too painful before). After ten sessions, Meaghan bought her own AO Scan Digital Body Analyzer. Her health continued to improve with nutritional and emotional support from Inner Voice.

Meaghan says that in addition to the support she received from the AO Scanner, the ThetaChamber℠ *has also* helped tremendously with anxiety relief and relieving unbearable pain. Her treatments at Theta Wellness Center gave her more stamina, and now she is high on life!

Insomnia

Insomnia, trouble initiating or maintaining sleep, is a common sleep disorder. Sleep disorders are common: over 70 million Americans are affected each year. The Cleveland Clinic defines people with Insomnia as those who can't fall asleep or stay asleep or who wake up too early. They will often wake up still feeling tired. Insomnia can affect not only your mood and energy level but also your overall health (diabetes, hypertension, and weight gain), work performance, lack of concentration or memory, and quality of life.

Approximately 33-55% of the world's adult population experiences insomnia at any given time. Chronic Insomnia Disorder, associated with stress or impairment, is estimated in 10-15% of those. By definition, short-term insomnia lasts days or weeks and is often caused by stress. Long-term insomnia is when sleep disturbance occurs at least three times per week for three months or longer.

There are many environmental, physiological, and psychological factors that can contribute to the development of insomnia. These can include life stressors (job, relationships, financial difficulties, etc.), unhealthy lifestyle or sleep habits, chronic diseases or pain, anxiety disorders or mental health challenges, hormone fluctuations, medication or other substances, neurological disorders (Alzheimer's disease, Parkinson's disease), and sleep disorders.

> *"Lack of sleep is only bad if you have to drive, or think, or talk, or move."*
>
> \- Dov Davidoff

Anyone who has suffered from sleeplessness knows it is not fun. There is an anonymous quote that says, "I want to sleep, but my mind won't stop talking to itself." We read a meme that well-depicts the cycle of one suffering from insomnia:

> Morning: Tired
> Afternoon: Dying for a Rest
> Evening: Can't Sleep

Sleep is the only sedentary activity that is *good* for you. Experts typically recommend a minimum of seven hours of sleep nightly for adults. Currently, only 59% of U.S. adults meet the minimum seven hours of slumber. But in 1942, 85% did. It's been said that if you fix your sleep, you will fix just about every other area of your life.

In addition to the frustration of not being rested, sleep deprivation is now being linked to physical breakdown: type-2 diabetes, obesity, cardiovascular problems, and compromised immune response. Treating the underlying cause can resolve insomnia. Our program provides different modalities to support you in obtaining a restful night's sleep. Our Insomnia program incorporates some of the following equipment:

ThetaChamber℠: synchronizes neural pathways, reduces stress hormones, and resets brainwaves.

AO Scan Digital Body Analyzer: includes comprehensive full body scan, and vitals report, and supports balanced emotions with optimizing tones.

Hyperbaric Chamber: low-pressure hyperbaric oxygen improves blood flow and increases oxygen saturation. Optional within the hyperbaric chamber are the acoustic light wave and an oxygen concentrator.

rTMS: promotes sleep-related hormones, synchronizes neural pathways, promotes hippocampal neurogenesis, and stimulates brain cells.

At a recent conference for Wounded Blue, we were privileged to bring the Tune-Up Station (a mobile Inner Voice unit) to use the Inner Voice feature for many of the attendees. The greatest common thread among those who participated was an inability to go to sleep, stay asleep, or both. Because the conference was over several days, we were able to get feedback from those who had an Inner Voice scan and received and played their balancing tones. One participant said that after having their Inner Voice scanned, they went to their room and took a long, hard nap during the afternoon. It had been 20 years since he had been able to nap, and he felt very rested. He then replayed his balancing tones and went back to sleep. (He couldn't remember the last time he was able to rest peacefully.) Others at the conference who had utilized an Inner Voice scan commented that after listening to their tones, they, too, were able to get to sleep, stay asleep, and get a great evening rest.

Attention Deficit Disorder (ADD), Attention Deficit Hyperactivity Disorder (ADHD) & Oppositional Defiant Disorder (ODD)

ADD and ADHD are medical conditions that can begin in childhood and persist into adulthood, contribute to low self-esteem, troubled relationships, difficulty at school, at work, and in relationships. They reflect a deficiency in a neurotransmitter called norepinephrine along with lower levels of dopamine which carry signals between nerves in the brain. This condition can affect attention, the ability to sit still, self-control, impulsivity, or the persistent repetition of words, actions, and behaviors.

Attention Deficit Disorder (ADD) is an older term for what is now known as the inattentive type of Attention Deficit Hyperactivity Disorder (ADHD). Since 1994, doctors have used the term to describe both inattentive and hyperactive types. Many parents, teachers, and adults continue to use the term ADD as a way to indicate the condition does not include the symptom of hyperactivity. ADHD is a neurological disorder that causes a range of behavior problems, such as difficulties with paying attention to instruction, focusing on tasks, keeping up with assignments, completing tasks, and social interactions.

Oppositional Defiant Disorder (ODD) is a behavior condition in which the child displays a continuing pattern of uncooperative, defiant, and sometimes hostile behavior toward people in authority. The majority of children and teens who have been diagnosed with ODD also have at least one other mental health condition including ADHD, anxiety disorders (including obsessive-compulsive disorder (OCD)), learning difficulties, mood disorders (such as depression,) and impulse control disorders. Around 40% of children who have ADHD have also been diagnosed with ODD. We offer the following equipment to help support those with ADD, ADHD, and ODD:

ThetaChamber℠: synchronizes neural pathways, reduces stress hormones, and synchronizes brainwaves.

rTMS: increases serotonin and dopamine, synchronizes neural pathways, and stimulates brain cells.

LED Light Bed: reduces emotional stress, activates endorphins, and balances the thalamus and hypothalamus.

Vibe Plate: increases circulation, enhances blood flow, and reduces stress hormones.

AO Scan is recommended as it provides whole body health status and balances emotions.

Charley's Story
The guardians of Charley, a ten-year-old, brought him to the Theta Wellness Center because they didn't know where else to go. He had been diagnosed with ODD (in addition to ADHD), and

it broke their hearts to see his struggle. They put him on a one-month protocol, and after the first week, they already saw amazing changes happening. One day Charley explained that he could tell there was a change deep in his core, and he felt really good. He went through a lot of emotional traumas the following several months but was now better able to think things through, have more self-control, and do much better. His guardians report he is not the same kid! The Theta Way gave them all hope and change they never thought possible.

Executive Tune-Up

The working environment has changed for many Americans, creating escalated stress levels. Seven in ten executives struggle to maintain a healthy work-life balance. Studies reveal that executives who are stressed over time experience physical, emotional, or mental exhaustion. It is important to recognize job-induced stress and learn how to process it. The executive tune-up enhances memory and focus by up to 24% while reducing stress and anxiety. Some of the following equipment is included in our Executive Tune-Up program:

ThetaChamber℠: synchronizes neural pathways, reduces stress hormones, and resets brainwaves.

LED Light Bed: reduces emotional stress, activates endorphins, and balances the thalamus and hypothalamus.

rTMS: increases serotonin and dopamine, synchronizes neural pathways, and stimulates brain cells.

AO Scan Digital Body Analyzer: includes comprehensive full body scan, and vitals report, and supports balanced emotions with optimizing tones.

Jon's Story

While in a high-level position in upper management, Jon, 43, experienced a close personal loss. This resulted in sleepless nights and an inability to turn off his brain. He had already developed some bad lifestyle choices as a way to cope with the stress and anxiety of his job. He felt he was physically and mentally at a tipping point (not in a good way) when he came through our doors. After completing an Executive Tune-Up program, he was able to sleep better, had less anxiety and stress, and had begun making some beneficial lifestyle changes. Jon reported that his performance at work had improved, the stress of the job was not daunting to him, and overall, he felt more effective and productive.

Neuropathy

Neuropathy is a nerve problem that causes pain, numbness, tingling, swelling, or muscle weakness in the hands or feet and can get worse over time. Peripheral neuropathy indicates a problem within the peripheral nervous system, a network of nerves outside your brain and spinal cord. Peripheral neuropathy can result from traumatic injuries, infections, metabolic problems, kidney failure, chronic alcoholism, exposure to toxins, autoimmune diseases, and commonly, diabetes.

Typical treatments involve physical therapy, over-the-counter painkillers, or prescriptions. Our neuropathy protocol includes:

RF Inner Cleanse: improve blood circulation, breaks up energy blockages, and opens meridians.

LED Light Bed: reduces emotional stress, activates endorphins, and balances the thalamus and hypothalamus.

Vibe Plate: increases circulation, enhances blood flow, and reduces stress hormones.

AO Scan is recommended as it provides whole body health status and supports balanced emotions.

Pain Management

Pain can become debilitating and frustrating, and interfere with sleep, work, family time, and daily activity. Pain, acute or chronic, can affect you physically and emotionally.

Pain is a general term that described uncomfortable sensations in the body. People feel pain when a signal travels through nerve fibers to the brain for interpretation involving both the mind and body. Mind-body therapies are more effective in alleviating pain by changing the way your brain perceives it. We incorporate some of the following equipment into our Pain Management programs:

ThetaChamber℠: synchronizes neural pathways, reduces stress hormones, and resets brainwaves.

LED Light Bed: anti-inflammatory, reduces pain, reduces stress, balances nerves.

Hyperbaric Chamber: low-pressure hyperbaric improves blood flow, increases oxygen levels, synchronizes neural pathways, and improves focus, concentration, and memory. Optional within the hyperbaric chamber are the acoustic light wave and an oxygen concentrator.

rTMS: increases serotonin and dopamine, improves concentration, increases memory, synchronizes neural pathways, and stimulates brain cells.

Bill's Story

Bill, age 78, could hardly walk when he came to us. He had worked in construction all of his life and the harsh demands of the job had created chronic pain, with decreased function mobility in his lower legs, feet, and hands. He had officially been diagnosed with neuropathy by his physician. He had done research on the medications (and side effects) the doctor wanted to prescribe to him, and Bill was seeking an alternative to medicine. He completed a program in which he used the Vibe Plate and RF (for neuropathy), and the LED Light Bed and Hyperbaric Chamber to decrease the inflammation. After each treatment, he noted a continuous improvement in his mobility and a decrease in pain.

Concentration, Focus, & Memory

Strong focus, memory, and concentration depend on the health and vitality of your brain. Whether you are a student studying for exams, a working professional interested in doing all you can to stay mentally sharp, or just looking to preserve and enhance your mental performance, non-invasive technology can help.

The human brain has an astonishing ability to adapt and change. With the right stimulation, your brain can form new neural pathways and alter existing connections to enhance your ability to learn new information and improve your memory at any age.

Theta Wellness Center provides different modalities to support you in strengthening your mental performance. Protocol includes:

ThetaChamber[SM]: synchronizes neural pathways, reduces stress hormones, and resets brainwaves.

LED Light Bed: anti-inflammatory, reduces pain, reduces stress, and balances nerves.

Hyperbaric Chamber: low-pressure hyperbaric improves blood flow and increases oxygen saturation. Optional within the hyperbaric chamber are the acoustic light wave and an oxygen concentrator.

AO Scan Digital Body Analyzer: includes comprehensive full body scan, and vitals report, and supports balanced emotions with optimizing tones.

Edith's Story
Edith, 75, was suffering from worsening dementia. She would get severely agitated about not being able to remember simple things or complete daily tasks, which was becoming very stressful for the family. She began a one-month program (2 times per week), utilizing the Hyperbaric Chamber, ThetaChamber℠, and LED Light Bed. After eight sessions, she reported that her memory had improved, and she was able to focus and complete tasks that used to unnerve her.

Students who utilize the ThetaChamber℠ prior to big tests tell us they believe it helped them to destress, focus and have better memory and concentration during testing.

Athletic Edge

You can improve your athletic edge through neuroscience. Our ThetaChamber℠ technology has been shown to improve mental concentration and enhance motor skills. Our equipment can help reduce stress hormones, reset brain waves, balance nerves, increases oxygen levels, reduce inflammation, and help improve focus.

We use a drug-free, scientific, neurological approach that supports health and wellness while improving your brain and body performance. To support you and help you get an edge on your performance, we offer:

> **ThetaChamber**[SM]: synchronizes neural pathways, reduces stress hormones, and resets brainwaves.
>
> **LED Light Bed**: anti-inflammatory, reduces healing time, stimulates ATP, increases collagen, and reduces stress, balances nerves.
>
> **Hyperbaric Chamber**: low-pressure hyperbaric increases oxygen levels and improves workout recovery and healing time. Optional within the hyperbaric chamber are the acoustic light wave and an oxygen concentrator.
>
> **Hydrogen Therapy**: anti-inflammatory, reduces oxidative stress.

Greg's Story

Greg, age 49, an avid golfer, participated regularly in a number of tournaments throughout the year. He was gifted a spin in the ThetaChamber[SM], which he used prior to an upcoming golf tournament. The Chamber settings were for anti-stress, anxiety, memory, focus, and concentration. After 30 minutes, he felt relaxed and more mentally ready to compete. He reported that it upped his game, and he placed top three in the tournament.

Boosted Immunity

A strong immune system gives you an edge on staying healthy and fighting off infections, illness, and disease. Over 80 autoimmune disorders are caused by immune system problems that cause inflammation.

If your immune system starts attacking instead of safeguarding your body, you are open to bacteria, viruses, and parasites, or could develop an autoimmune disorder. Our technology boosts your immunity using the following equipment:

ThetaChamber℠: synchronizes neural pathways and reduces stress hormones.

LED Light Bed: anti-inflammatory, antibacterial, stimulates immunity.

Hyperbaric Chamber: low-pressure hyperbaric increases oxygen levels and improves immune cell response. Optional within the hyperbaric chamber are the acoustic light wave and an oxygen concentrator.

Hydrogen Therapy: antioxidant, anti-inflammatory, reduces oxidative stress.

Liz's Story

Liz, 71, went on a trip last year and, within the week, was very ill. Blood tests ordered by her doctor determined that her liver was not functioning properly, and she had a viral infection. She had no energy and was almost unable to get out of bed. Her blood work showed Liz's iron count was extremely low. In fact, her doctor told her to go directly to the ER for a blood transfusion. Instead, she immediately got on iron supplements and looked for an alternative to a transfusion. She used the Hyperbaric chamber with Acoustic Light Wave (set on virus), and the LED Light Bed (set at 584 HZ for liver assistance). She also began working with a naturopath taking recommended supplements to build up her blood iron. Liz says she feels back to her old self and continues on a recommended maintenance plan.

Whole Body Detox

Detoxing is about cleansing, nourishing, and resting your body from the inside out. Today we are exposed to more toxins in our environment and food sources than ever before. The body has a very sophisticated way of eliminating toxins that involve the liver, kidneys, digestive system, skin, lungs, intestines, bowels, and lymphatic system.

Toxins can impede a body's natural defense. Whole body detox is a way to eliminate toxins, improve your health, improve blood circulation, and promote weight loss. The following equipment is included in our Detox programs:

RF Inner Cleanse: improves blood circulation, eliminates toxins, detoxes organs, and increases metabolism.

LED Light Bed: stimulates ATP, increases collagen production, and reduces inflammation.

Hyperbaric Chamber: low-pressure hyperbaric improves blood flow and increases oxygen levels. Optional within the hyperbaric chamber are the acoustic light wave and an oxygen concentrator.

Vibe Plate: increases circulation, enhances blood flow, and stimulates the lymphatic system.

AO Scan is recommended as it provides whole body health status and supports balanced emotions.

Caleb's Story
Caleb, 27, wanted to give up vaping and alcohol. His job required that he drive long distances from client to client, which caused him to spend a lot of time on the road. He used vaping to help pass the time of long hours on the road. He used alcohol

at the end of his workday to calm the stress of being on the road with "crazy" drivers all day. He completed a 21-day program which included the ThetaChamber[SM] (set to tobacco, alcohol, stress/anxiety), the rTMS, and the LED Light Bed. During his program, he was also provided nutrition support that included smoothies with supplements to support the liver (detoxification and conjugation) and other organs of elimination. Caleb reports that he has been able to change his unwanted habits and no longer has cravings.

Tune-Up Station

Negative emotions and unprocessed stress can put your health in jeopardy. There is not an identified age group that is affected more than another; all ages and professions have felt the changes taking place in the world in which we live. Wouldn't it be wonderful if, instead of taking a pill (with side effects) to make you feel better, you could spend a few minutes a day and "tune up" your emotional bearings? That is possible.

A Tune-Up station is a new concept developed by Theta Wellness Center utilizing Inner Voice brain science to unlock the door to stress, anxiety, depression, and the emotions that eventually lead to dis-ease. Inner Voice technology uses sound harmonizing techniques, which generate balanced audio frequencies. These balanced frequencies can counter those that are in excess and supplement frequencies that are lacking.

Your voice is recorded for 20 seconds then analyzed to determine your current emotional state. Inner Voice focuses on four frequencies: three notes that are excessively out of balance (over-compensated), and one note that is being suppressed.

Sound harmonizing tones are generated to support and balance your emotional and mental states. Four audio files are sent to you that correspond to each of the zones received in your report. The more you listen to the tones, the better the results.

A Tune-Up station is mobile and can be used in schools, public agencies, businesses, and organizations. It provides a place for people of all ages to rebalance their emotional state of being and reduce their stress and anxiety while improving concentration, creativity, and emotional intelligence. The modality includes the AO Scan Inner Voice that can be used anytime, anywhere.

"You are what you eat, so don't be fast, easy, cheap, or fake."
- Unknown

7 HEALTH BEGINS IN THE GUT

Why the Gut is so Important

Hippocrates was accurate in saying, "Health begins in the gut." Several body functions are affected by the ability of the gut (gastrointestinal tract) to be balanced, healthy, and functioning at an optimum level. Neurologists refer to our gut as our second brain because nearly 80% of our immune system is located in the gut. As many neurotransmitters are produced in the gut as in the brain: 85-90% of the "feel good" hormone, serotonin, as well as the production of norepinephrine, dopamine, and melatonin. Your gut health is important to your overall well-being.

Many people are familiar with the term "leaky gut" yet don't realize that they may be well on their way to having a full-blown case of it. Foods today are not what they were even a few decades ago. The nutritional value of food is suffering. Sugar level consumption is at an all-time high. Gluten sensitivity has massively increased, and the use of unhealthy or rancid oils that compromise the gut is widespread.

These conditions can cause the lining of the gut to develop small holes that allow food particles to enter the bloodstream and produce an immune response. Symptoms can include gas, bloating, constipation, or a host of other gut-related issues.

People, often unaware they have gut problems because they don't feel sick or bloated, assume all is well. They may have even questioned their doctor or health practitioner and been told their gut is fine. Symptoms may not even show up in the gut but possibly as depression, anxiety, brain fog, skin issues, weight gain, joint aches, or systemic inflammation.

Changes in personality, anger, depression, or anxiety can be more clues that the body is not properly digesting. Looking at what you are eating and drinking can be important to solving many of these challenging issues. Food lists can provide clues, which is one of the reasons a comprehensive allergy list is incorporated into the Vitals report of our clients' AO Digital Body Scans.

Problems with the Standard American Diet

The average American's diet consists of excess sodium, saturated fats, refined carbohydrates, calories from solid fats, and added sugars. These foods are passed through drive-through windows, ordered on an app, delivered to our doors, and found in the local grocery store in cans, boxes, bottles, and in the freezer section. It is estimated that 63% of America's calories come from refined and processed foods, many of which have no true nutrients and wreak havoc on the health of millions of Americans.

Additionally, modern farming practices don't help the problem. We have been genetically modifying foods for years, over-farming land, and using multiple chemicals as fertilizers and preservatives. As it gets digested, along with our food, the result has been chronic health-related issues on the rise.

The current allopathic healthcare system is a crisis-care system. While doctors are trained to deal with crises, they are not necessarily trained to deal with health. Therefore, they may offer prescription medications and surgeries for many health-related problems without first asking about simple daily health habits and nutrition. There is a growing awareness that medicine is not the answer to everything.

We recently learned of an adolescent girl who started having seizures. After much medical testing and several medical scans, she was put on anti-seizure medicine but continued to have seizures. Through work with a Naturopath, she stopped eating gluten, soy, and grains. Within three months of her new dietary regimen, she stopped having seizures. After six months of eating this way, she continued to be seizure-free, so her doctor took her off the prescribed anti-seizure medicine.

"The food you eat can be either the safest and most powerful form of medicine or the slowest form of poison."

– Ann Wigmore

Other Causes of Poor Gut Health

Healing the gut begins with asking the right questions and investigating what is behind the symptoms of poor health. Toxins in the environment, chemicals, pesticides, mold, fungus, parasites, viruses, bacteria, and food can play a part in disrupting the gut, as well as the following:

Hydration can be a major issue. To say water is an essential nutrient for your body and health is an understatement. Dehydrated people not only suffer health and elimination problems, but they also walk around like a big piece of beef jerky. It's estimated that 60-75% of your body is made up of water; it is the essential fluid of life. You can survive three weeks without food but only three days without water. Water keeps the muscles moving, cleans the body, curbs overeating, and is good for your brain. It is not just a transport system but an actual nutrient that affects every function in the body and is a major component of brain function.

Lack of water affects the gut in a number of ways. Constipation is a major repercussion, affecting the integrity of the gut and the entire health of the body. What goes in must come out, so healthy elimination is important. A healthy stool is typically brown in color; a normal bowel movement is one that occurs between two times a day and three times a week. If you are experiencing more or less, you might want to pay attention to that.

The large intestine absorbs a lot of the body's electrolytes, uses fiber to produce vitamins, and produces the majority of your serotonin. About 40 of your 100 neurotransmitters needed for mental and physical health are produced in the gut. This ability is majorly affected by dehydration, and unfortunately, many people are chronically dehydrated without realizing it. How much water do you need? The general rule of thumb is to drink at least half your body weight in ounces. For example, a 140-pound person should consume about 70+ ounces of water per day.

Not all beverages are created equal. The population, to a large degree, has replaced water with soda, coffee, energy drinks, and alcohol, which don't count as water. They are molecularly different and actually steal water from the body. Drinks with caffeine cause the body to excrete more water. Sugary drinks, such as juice and soda, can rob water from the intestines, which reduces the health of your body and offers none of the benefits that water by itself provides. When you do drink water, the quality of that water is another consideration: tap water has a lot of ingredients that can compromise health. Investigate your water source. Drinking filtered, clean water is a key to good health.

Emotion is a major affecter of gut health. The brain releases peptides into the bloodstream in response to emotion, and the peptides can affect the different organs, glands, and systems to the point that their function is reduced or there is an inflammatory response. Many of the diseases a person would seek a doctor's help for involve inflammation.

The adrenals produce stress hormones necessary for life. If their need for minerals is high, the rest of the body gets robbed. The result is reduced acid production by the stomach, reduced enzymes for the duodenum, where the food is prepared for the rest of the gut, and reduced lymphatic ability to function, causing reduced hormone functioning. These dis-functions create food fermentation and gut lining aggravation on a daily basis.

Stress and anxiety are among the most important contributors to poor gut function. Leakiness of the gut walls allows different materials to get into the blood and wreak major problems, such as autoimmune disease. According to the National Institute of Environmental Sciences, more than 24 million Americans suffer from an autoimmune disease. That is more than 7% of the population. An additional eight million people have auto-antibodies, blood molecules that indicate a person's chance of developing autoimmune disease.

Parasites can be another issue. When the diet is high in sugar, high fructose corn syrup, and gluten, lack of nutrients, full of pesticides, and is low in nutrition, the gut becomes an ideal environment for parasites. They like to hang out in the "fine dining section" of the gut by the pancreas and the ducts that lead up to the liver and gall bladder. They compete for your nutrition, and the result can be a lot of toxicity in the body. It is very common for people to have parasites. They lurk in the soil, contaminated food and water, uncooked or undercooked meat, and unclean fruits and vegetables, and they are easily passed on. Doing a parasite cleanse once or twice per year is usually a good idea for most people.

The Brain-Gut Connection

The blood-brain barrier (BBB) is composed of many cell types that provide a structural, functional roadblock to bacteria, viruses, fungi, parasites, chemicals, heavy metals, and other pathogens, but allow small particles in and out as necessary. A compromised gut can cause the BBB to become leaky, like the gut. When harmful substances are able to pass through the walls and find their way into the brain, it can change the way you function every day. Unwanted substances entering the brain can cause brain inflammation, which, over time, can damage and destroy brain tissue and accelerate brain degeneration.

A leaky brain can be linked to brain fog, difficulty concentrating, headaches, migraines, sleep issues, depression, ADD/ADHD, chronic pain, autism, cognitive impairment, Alzheimer's, parkinson's disease, seizures, facial palsies, schizophrenia, and other mental illnesses.

According to Dr. Kristien Boyle, a leaky brain can be caused by a bad diet, poor digestion, antioxidant status, head trauma, unstable/high blood sugar, vitamin B deficiency, heavy metals, gluten, chronic stress, chronic or systemic inflammation, leaky gut, and a host of other problems. And, he notes, a diet full of soda or energy drinks, processed snacks, and fast food doesn't help either.[30]

The list of leaky brain causes and symptoms may seem long, but the good news is there are a number of things you can do to help heal a leaky blood-brain barrier. First and foremost, heal your leaky gut. Leaks in both places happen for the same reasons. Focusing on healing the gut often resolves symptoms of a leaky brain.

Metals, Molds, Pollutants, & Pesticides

Just as with food modification and additives, these pervasive toxins and their effects are more far-reaching than most people are aware. For example, interruption of hormone balance, brain fog, inability to lose weight, anger and rage, depression, chronic immune system challenges, chronic brain challenges, and insomnia can often be linked to high levels of any combination of metals, molds, pollutants, or pesticides. When we do comprehensive AO Digital Body Analyzer scans, it has become increasingly common to find high levels of toxicities in the body.

In traditional medicine, doctors don't always look at heavy metals because, typically, there isn't a medicine to prescribe that will "fix" it. The methods they do use, such as intravenous chelation, can be harsh. Dumping a bunch of heavy metals into the system of a very ill person can be too much for the body to handle and can cause a healing crisis.

---

[30] Dr. Boyle D.A.C.M., Lac, Kipi OM, https://www.holisticcharlotte.com/do-you-have-a-leaky-brain-perform-this-test-to-find-out/Stress Gut Link, June 29, 2017

"People do not decide their futures; they decide their habits, and their habits decide their future."
– F.M. Alexander

Jeff's Story

Jeff, 48, had been living in a dank house built in New England in the 1800s. His AO Digital Body Analyzer Scan showed he was full of mold and fungus. In addition, his job exposed him daily to mold and fungus as he was required to clear out warehouses. To support him in his fight against mold and fungus, we put Jeff on a nutritional plan which included increasing amino acids, reducing sugar, a brain food supplement, greens and fruits, and a high dose of niacin. He additionally utilized the AO Digital Body Analyzer Scan, Acoustic Light Wave, and hydrogen breathing treatments. After three weeks, he retested, and there was a substantial reduction in the presence of mold. He also noticed the brain fog he had been experiencing was gone.

The Benson Family's Story

The Benson family came to us, having returned to the mainland after living on a tropical island for over ten years. The father, mother, and daughter all tested positive for parasites, mold, and fungus. Their health complaints included having no energy, tiring easily, brain fog, and the mother had severe anemia. They completed a 21-day program utilizing diet changes, Acoustic Light Wave, Hyperbaric Chamber, LED Light Bed, and, to help with emotions, the ThetaChamber[SM]. After, all three reported feeling great: restored energy, a sense of good health, clear thinking, better color, and no digestion or depression issues.

We Offer Resources that can Educate and Aid You in Your Healing Journey:

Negative Ion H₂O Sticks

Hydration is one of the easiest, cheapest steps you can take to improve your health. Negative Ion H2O Sticks can help you reach your hydration goals. Plan to drink 50% (aim for 75%) of your weight in ounces, up to a gallon a day. Start early in the day and finish by about 6 PM to not interfere with sleep. Remember that coffee, tea (unless herbal), and soda do not count. If you are someone who either doesn't like the taste of water or doesn't trust what's in the water you drink, we offer Negative Ion H2O Sticks. The high-intensity Tourmaline and Si Bin ceramic beads minimize and energize the water molecules to increase absorption and elimination of the water in the body. They also neutralize bacteria, serve as an antioxidant, help minimize the absorption of glucose and improve the absorption of minerals from food. Our clients report they make their water taste better, and have a smoother texture.

ThetaChamber℠

Find a Theta Wellness Center near you for access to the ThetaChamber℠. The ThetaChamber℠ is unique in its ability to help with digestion and gut health. The combination of the modalities encompassed in its programs is able to address the root causes of many of the gut-brain axis issues. Forging new healthy pathways sidesteps a lot of the time involved in trying to support health issues through other methods, such as meditation or reestablishing gut health through supplements alone.

One major benefit of utilizing the ThetaChamber℠ is the ability of the stomach to now utilize minerals to produce acid and pepsin and the endocrine system to produce gastrin that promotes and is actively involved with the stomach making acid and pepsin. The resulting proper breakdown of food can have a profound effect on the health of your body. The Theta-Chamber℠ supports you in healing the gut so you can heal the body. The gut-brain connection is huge, so helping this all-important connection is crucial.

The ThetaChamber℠ can also help you address fear, anger, depression, addiction, hormone balance, focus, and concentration. This matters because digestion is greatly impacted by the Vagus nerve and the sympathetic-para-sympathetic relationship in the body. And the adrenals are directly affected; reducing their stress level allows additional trace minerals to be available to all nine body systems.

AO Digital Body Analyzer Scan

Next, consider having an in-depth scan at the center by means of an AO Digital Body Scan. The scanner can assist your brain in making better selections regarding the foods you may be sensitive to and provide information on your body regarding the presence of mold, fungus, heavy metals, bacteria, viruses, pesticides, chemicals, emotions, allergens, genetic miasms (predispositions), parasites, and other categories.

In restoring gut and brain health, having access to revealing and relevant information about your body – an owner's manual of sorts – can be very helpful. The AO Digital Body Scan is a unique educational tool that can help you learn about how your body is performing. It provides a timely, safe, simple, non-invasive way for you to collect the information you need to make life-altering decisions about your brain and gut health.

Inner Voice

With Inner Voice, your voice is recorded, then analyzed to determine your current emotional state. The technology focuses on three notes that are excessively out of balance (overcompensated), as well as one note that is being suppressed. Sound harmonizing tones are generated and emailed to support you in balancing your emotional and mental states. Stress impacts every part of your body, from digestion to your immune system. It can lead to higher cortisol levels that can stimulate appetite and cravings for unhealthy food choices. Playing your optimizing tones when stressed, anxious, or emotional can help bring you to a state of balance.

Vitals Scan

The Vitals Scan mode of the AO Digital Body Scan quickly performs a complete scan of every bodily function with an analysis. Utilizing a transducer headset, the AO Digital Body Scan communicates with the body via subtle bio-frequencies and electromagnetic signals to identify the areas that may need assistance. This provides you with a concise snapshot of the blueprint frequencies in relationship to the frequencies produced by the blood, organs, glands, and systems of the body.

The Scan produces reports on the following systems: blood, chakra, gastrointestinal, meridian, nutritional, physical functionality, and toxicities.

Comprehensive Scan

The Comprehensive Scan provides a complete and thorough system status snapshot with optimization of hundreds of blueprint frequencies associated with nine body systems.

This scan identifies areas in need of support. Each system report is designed to educate you about areas of possible cause and offers suggestions to improve your overall health. Body systems scanned include circulation, connective tissue, musculoskeletal, digestion, endocrine, lymphatic, nervous, respiratory sensory nervous, integumentary, urinary, human cell, and mitochondria.

"The purpose of life after all, is to live it, to taste experience to the utmost, to reach out eagerly and without fear for newer and richer experience."

― Eleanor Roosevelt

ACKNOWLEDGMENTS

This book is a product of the contributions of several people whose input we greatly appreciate. First, thank you to Teresa Cone, M.D., Cathy Lamar, Amber Venzke, and Dennis Dohner for taking the time to read through the writing phases and guiding us on what may be more easily understood. Jaime Partlow is the brains and creativity behind the cover art.

We are grateful to Loran Swensen, INNERgy Development, LLC, www.innergydev.com, for generously sharing with us his vision, ingenuity, and abundant knowledge of brain-body science. He has pioneered the theta technology modalities utilized at the Theta Wellness Center, and his dedication to bettering technology for health, wellness, and the best possible outcome for others is inspiring. A shout out to Heather Kellogg for generously sharing her experience in the health and wellness industry and for cheering us on.

Big thanks to Deborah Bruce of Amazone Health & Wellness, www.amazonehealth.com, for her help and support along the way. Like Loran, she has been involved in the use, development, and application of Inner Voice and programs that utilize theta science and frequency for quite some time. She knows her stuff and has helped many using theta technology.

The Theta Way

ABOUT THE AUTHORS

Janet Garland is the owner and director of Theta Wellness Center in Gold River, California. A lifelong entrepreneur, she is not new to the business world. In addition to cottage industry businesses that she started and grew to success in her earlier years, Janet is also a licensed contractor who has owned and run her own construction company since 2003.

Janet comes from a family with a medical background, in which she was strongly encouraged to pursue a medical career. During her education to become a nurse, she found herself drawn to business courses along the way. Not only has she used those skills in her own businesses, but has been involved in benevolent and civic organizations that focus on the betterment of underserved communities.

Janet lives in Sacramento, California, with her husband, Gary. They have two sons and two grandchildren.

Kristine Dohner has been ordained as a pastor since 2011, is certified in Brainspotting Trauma Therapy, and holds a degree in counseling. For over 22 years, she has taught and counseled people toward healing and wholeness in life and relationships. Her desire is that each person would be empowered and equipped to live in the fullness of their best possible life.

Kristine has also been involved in local government and is passionate about making a difference in her city and region.

She lives in Roseville, California, with her husband, Dennis, with whom she has co-authored *21 Days of ThanksLiving, Finding Your Joy at Christmas, Finding Your Peace, Got Jesus. Now What?*, and, soon to be released, *Finding Your Freedom*. They have seven children and eight grandchildren.

The Theta Way

Theta Wellness Center

11211 Gold Country Blvd. Suite 100

Gold River, California 95670

916-226-1940

www.thetawellnesinc.com

Made in the USA
Columbia, SC
11 September 2024